THE ART OF LIFE IS THE AVOIDING OF PAIN

Wilder Publications, Inc.
PO Box 632
Floyd VA 24091

ISBN 10: 1-61720-847-7
ISBN 13: 978-1-61720-847-8

First Edition

10 9 8 7 6 5 4 3 2 1

THE ART OF LIFE IS THE AVOIDING OF PAIN

by Brian Walters

CONTENTS

Hippocrates Never Traveled these Roads

Snowflakes in a Warm Hand

HIPPOCRATES NEVER TRAVELED THESE ROADS

HOME HEALTH

There are more than a dozen of us, sitting around three tables
discussing at the Tuesday morning team management meeting
the typical scenarios we discuss each week: Mrs. Blanks, half-blind, tripped
on a shoe while stepping out of bed, broke her pelvis, surgery,
in intensive care for at least a fortnight; Mr. Traterro,
emphysema, dementia, slipped on ice on his patio
after the last storm, fractured hip, needs nursing, physical therapy,
and a social worker to prepare the family for eventual hospice;
Mr. Packard, Alzheimer's, Parkinson's, unable to ambulate,
belligerent the previous time he needed health care
but his wife insists, to help him gain some semblance of independence;
Mrs. Peasoner, complains of nausea when standing
for more than 10 minutes at a time, unable to cook
or do laundry without fear of falling, occasional diarrhea
with her medication; Mrs. Talley, partial R Leg amputee,
sleeps with nine cats on her sofa and will cuss you out
if you suggest changing the kitty litter box more than once a month;
There are others, most to be seen four to six weeks,
some longer, some shorter, some until a room
in an assisted living facility becomes vacant,
or we get news they are in the hospital. . .or worse.

STANDING ROOM ONLY

It's one of those homes where there's no place
hygienic enough to sit, and I hate
even putting my medical bag down.
Chairs, moldy and stained with dog drool,
mashed crumbs from decades (centuries?)
and probably piss and who knows what else.
The lampshades draped with dust
and the once-white carpet now the color
of coal. The stove covered
with blackened pans and the remains
of scrambled eggs leftover from yesterday morning.
Ashtrays jammed with cigarette butts in every room
and the tub and toilet soiled with—*best not to guess.*
Magazines everywhere, I note a *Sports Illustrated*
from 1988 and a *Life* from 1950.
"My Paw and Maw bought this house in 1927,"
my patient tells me. Left it to me when they passed on
and I've lived here ever since."
I'm not here to dispute what the word "lived" means,
or tell the old man he might be safer
in a retirement facility after his recent stroke.
I'm just here to help him sit up in bed
and stand so he can lift his feet
securely over the mildewed carpets
to reach his closet for clothes
and be able to reach the sink to wash
and the kitchen to cook
and hopefully bend his knees with good posture
to feed his scurvy mutt
that lies unmoving on a torn cushion
beside the front door
not barking once

the whole time I'm
here.

WHAT'S RIGHT IS WRONG

THERAPIST

I've been working with her for three weeks;
returning home after a month in the hospital
for a broken hip, she is still not able to walk,
not even with a new walker. A part of me
believes she can, physically—much of her problem
is depression, her daughter died last year,
and her son lives in Arkansas, and her
only human contact on a daily basis
are two caregivers who split the AM-PM shifts—
but another part knows she is slowly sliding
to the grave, and even wants to: she states
life holds no meaning for her. I try and tell her
summer is here and the tulips outside her window
are beautiful and life has not left her yet,
but she sadly smiles and says, "Young man,
just wait till you get old. . ."

PATIENT

I know the boy means well. He must think
I'm awfully crabby at times, not wanting to do
the exercises he shows me, not wanting to stand up
or walk from my wheelchair through the living room.
He says it's only a few feet, but a few feet
are like a few miles at this point. Oh, what's the use. . .
I can hardly chew regular food anymore,
my bowels don't cooperate, I wear diapers,
one eye's gone, I'm half-deaf, and my legs
tremble even when I sit. And I'm always *cold*. . .
The weather's 80 degrees, but I freeze

even with my sweater on and two blankets
covering from toes to chin. Lord, I won't last another winter. . .
This therapy's just a waste of time.

KNOTS

Today's diagnosis: a 35 year-old man with diabetes,
recent stroke, continual swelling in the ankles,
heart palpitations and dizziness with walking,
inability to dorsiflex his feet, depression,
currently takes five medications and dialysis
three times a week.
        I see instantly that progress
will be slow, overall improvement minimal.
He sits in a crumb-filled recliner half-asleep
from the double-dose of Tylenol he took
a half hour before. A partly eaten Big Mac
lies in a wrapper on the floor next to a milk shake
and two tootsie rolls unopened.
        He says
he is too weak to exercise, too worn out
from the dialysis done in the morning.
Complains of grinding knees and wanting
to throw up.
        "I nearly fell a few hours ago
going to the bathroom," he adds with a yawn.

I end up massaging his hamstrings and quadriceps
above the knees, his calves, his achilles.
He grimaces and groans, but tells me not to stop.

"No, it's not that bad," he shrugs. "I've had
worse pain. Take my wife, for instance.
We were married four years, have two
of the loveliest girls you can imagine, twins,
and now I don't even get to see them. . ."

I tell him I'm sorry to hear that, and try not

to let him know that I notice his tears.

"Yeah. . .they're seven now, and every time
I call no one answers the phone, or the ex-
says they're visiting the grand-folks,
or with friends, or in the bath, or sleeping.

They live in Baltimore, a six-hour drive"
—he points at his swollen feet—
"and with these I can no longer drive.
"I'm fucked in all ways!"

I don't answer, just massage the muscles
that feel like knots that can never be unwound.
When I finish he frowns.
                              "I'm sorry, man,
I didn't mean to throw all my garbage on you.
It's just. . .there aren't many people to talk to
these days. I'm either sitting here watching
soap operas or in the doctor's office.
It ain't much of a life. No, it's not life.
But. . .I guess it could be a lot shittier."

EXAGGERATING! NOT ME

I've been in nursing homes that make 5-star hotels shabby,
I've been in others that are dumping grounds for the dying
and deceased whose coffins have yet to be sealed.
The bad ones are overrun with uncaring staff,
small rooms frigid in the winter and sweat shops in the summer,
food even roaches run away from, smells
that leave you gagging as soon as you walk in.

Like everything else in America there is no uniformity,
only a cross-section of services segregated by money
or lack of it. The wealthy have everything, the poorest nothing.

A *solution*. . .I'm not the right person to ask.
I merely tend to the half-corpses and the few remaining
energetic souls who just. . .

                              might. . .

                                        last

another day, fortnight,
or. . .even a year.

HOME RUN

The speech therapist warned me of Milt's dementia.
Though. . .she didn't say to what degree.
His house is a gray ruin of a shack lodged between two
chicken pens and what seems to be an outhouse.
The driveway (if there ever was one) is a pond
filled in with last week's storms. I park, open the door,
splash one foot in the water and jump the other
to a patch of thick mud and nearly fall.
Somehow I hold on to my laptop and medical bag.
Two dirty miniature poodles bark at me
from behind the back yard fence.
I knock on the door; someone shouts at me, I enter.
A woman in a wheelchair eyes me with wariness.

"Who are you?" she asks.

"Don't you remember? I'm the therapist.
I called a while back to set up an appointment."

"Oh. . .you mean with Milton. Well, come on in,
he's in the kitchen eating his breakfast."

I glance at my watch: 1:30 in the afternoon.

Milton is white-haired, obese, barefoot, sitting at a table
in a sweat-stained tee-shirt and boxer's
slurping up what appears to be a cross
between yoghurt and horse gruel.

"Hi, I'm Brian," I say.

He looks at me, startled. Doesn't respond.

19

Half of his food is already on his tee-shirt,
the other half drooling down his mouth.

"He prefers to be called Milt," his wife pipes in.

I take his vitals, ask a few questions to his wife
about pain level, activity level, functional abilities
and how often he gets B12 shots.
She tells me he can still walk (a little at a time)
but often has trouble walking in the bathroom
and almost fell two nights ago.

I pat him on the shoulder, startling him again.

"Milt, if you don't mind, I'd like to see you walk
to the bathroom and back. I'll make sure
you won't fall. That's a promise."

Pulling out a gait-belt, I tie it around his waist securely.
The gruel drips on it but it's washable.

I ask Milt to stand. He opens his mouth:
only one front tooth and a few molars.

He squints his eyes at me.

"Who'd you say you was?"

I tell him.

"Brian. . .? I don't know anyone named Brian."

"I'm here to treat you. . .for *physical therapy.*"

Still sitting, he tries to focus on me. One of his eyes
has a cataract.

"I worked for the town of Radford for forty-two years."

"That's good, Milt. I'm certain they were proud to have you—"

"I used to play baseball."

"Yeah, baseball's a fun sport."

"I played outfield. One time I hit a home run.
You should have seen me running around those bases."

He hoops and hollers and his wife from the living room
glares at him.

"That's all he talks about—his job and baseball.
He ain't done either in God-knows how long. . ."

A few more minutes pass before I half pull him from the chair
and he wobbles, losing his balance. I steady him,
holding tightly to the belt.

"Alright, Milt, let's walk to the bathroom."

The bathroom is to the right of the kitchen
but he turns left, crouched over like a hunchback
sliding his legs in a slow, shuffling gait,
feet lifting no more than an inch.

"Milt, we need to turn the other way—behind you."

But he keeps on shuffling, eyes rolling
in the sockets like pinballs
as he scours the terrain. He reaches
the living room where his wife is watching
The Price is Right. She shakes her head.

"Now Milton, the man"—what's your name again?—"Brian,
wants you to head to the bathroom. You go on
and turn around!"

He does, but not completely. His bare lizard feet
carry him to another room, the bedroom.
I stay beside him, and when he reaches the bed
he sits, panting from the effort.

"Why don't you take a breather,
then we can walk back."

He squints his eyes again.

"Hey. . .ain't you that feller from Salem I got in a fight with.
That must have been thirty years ago."

"No, Milt, I'm not."

"You sure look like him."

"It was someone else."

"You're lying!" He shakes a fist at me and growls.

Then as suddenly drops the fist and blinks, puzzled.

"Did I tell you I worked for the town of Radford for 42 years."

I smile, nodding.

"I used to play baseball."

I nod again.

"I'm tired."

Then with a movement quicker than any
he showed earlier, Milt lies across the bed,
closes his eyes, is still.

"Milt, let's go back to the kitchen.

Milt. . . Milt, you're not sleeping are you—"

"Oh Lord, when he gets in that bed you can't
get him up for hours." His wife has wheeled herself
into the bedroom. Frowning, she says,
"You best come another day"—what'd you say
your name was—"Brian, yes, just come on by
another day. How often you fixing
on treating him?"

I tell her I'll have to check my schedule,
which I do back in the car: Milton Forbes,
3x a week for six weeks. I read it again
to make certain. Then try and remember
if I have a baseball glove at home.

BARBARIANS AT THE GATES OF ROME

"Unbelievable! He's only been here two weeks
and already his watch and ring have been stolen.
A $1200 gold watch; and the ring from Vanderbilt
when he received his Ph.D. He wouldn't take it off,
but now someone else has. . ."

The woman is near tears; I console her
with a few words and a kind nod. I have come
to the **Calm Fields** nursing home to treat her husband
for physical therapy. A victim of a stroke on the left side,
he lingers most days in bed unable to speak or hear,
and during the rare moments a sentence
leaves his tongue it is baby-garble
or the hallucinations of a soul in a world not ours.

His wife continues to vent her rage, threatening
to remove him from the facility, return him home.
But I look at her and she knows that I know
such a plan is beyond possibility.
Frail herself, and unable to keep him from falling
in the bathroom or anywhere in their house
for that matter, her wet eyes acknowledge
the truth that is so final.
                              I tell her from now on
never to allow valuables and mementos in his room.
The facility coordinators gave her the same advice
on Jon's admittance—the same advice they give everyone.
Theft happens, just like strokes and Parkinson's.
The sick and dying are out for themselves,
Nature is indifferent and the gods are silent.

THE LUCKY ONE

I cross the New River near Eggleston
where rock-ridges hug rhododendrons and blue violets
sway in breezes over the northward current.
Shawnee once fished the shallows here, and hunted
deer and elk in forests. Frontiersmen followed
on the worn paths, straying west. . .or staying.

The shallower runlets remain, but the woods
have been trimmed to accommodate cattle farms
and isolated churches and houses jetting smoke
from wood-burning stoves. In ten minutes I'll enter
such a house to treat a man who moved to these mountains
south from Cleveland desiring warmer winters and seclusion.

"Oh, I've had therapy before," he tells me, lifting up the stump
of his right leg with a grunt. He takes oxygen
through tubes in his nose—"Emphysema! All those packs
of cigarettes since I was twelve"—and regularly has heartburn.
"My wife's not doing too well either," he adds.
Despite all he says, his vitals are not bad—not *great*—but good

for someone who can barely breathe. I have him do knee
extensions in his wheelchair and he laughs. "As you can see,
I don't have much of a knee." Unaware of his history
I ask how he became an amputee. He shrugs, "Nam."
I don't ask further but he elaborates. "Tripped
on a hidden wire in a stream. Strange. . .I was one
of the lucky ones. Two other guys bought the farm."

His stump is raw, and red from recent infection.
"I take antibiotics," he states, "but the damned shit's not working.
If it keeps up like this the doc's going to remove

the rest of the leg." He looks at me as though I can provide
the answer. But it's not my job to gainsay the physician.

I do what I can, don't overpush him. His breaths come
in sobs after a few exercises, a few repetitions.
I massage his thigh briefly, but there is too much pain.

I tell him I'll come again Friday, just before noon.
"I'll be here," he says, "or in the mortuary."
And. . .as we lock eyes I half-believe him.

AND YOU'VE GIVEN TO ME

Then there are the happy stories. . .
Edna who fell down while feeding her chickens
was frightened of going outside for a month afterward
or even walking inside her house
until I made her believe she could start with a walker,
then a cane, and finally use her improved balance
and coordination from standing and stepping on a foam pad
to simulate ambulating on uneven ground and tufts of grass.
I watched her throw seed to her chickens as she smiled and said,
"Never thought I'd do this again."

And the tale of Timmy who was born with a withered left arm
and two unstable legs and succumbed to seizures
unhelped by medication. He wanted to walk normal
so I walked him over every surface level possible: wood floor,
soft rugs, concrete, gravel, grass, dirt, mud, up and down stairs,
frontwards, backwards, sideways, stepping over cups,
cones, logs, lawnmowers, puddles, dog poop.
When we discharged him he shook my hand and nearly cried. . .
"I'm doing stuff I've only dreamed about."

And C.H. who hurt a disk lifting motors at the local auto plant
while falling and breaking a femur. He wanted to return to work
so I pushed him when he moaned that seated leg lifts were like
        knives in the knee,
I pushed him to use his crutches when he didn't want
to rise from his chair, I pushed him to use one crutch,
then. . .no crutch, I pushed him to stand on one foot
and hold it for thirty seconds, I pushed him to walk fast: stop:
walk slow, I pushed him till he said under his breath
that I was a son of bitch, I pushed him till he gripped my shoulder
on the last day and was short of words:
"Man. . .you've given me my life back."

YOU CAN ONLY SHUT THE DRAWBRIDGE SO LONG

It's not enough that I have to drive up dirt-road mountains
and through dilapidated trailer parks to treat people
who can barely walk, or can't walk, are stooped over
and diabetic, need oxygen tanks to breathe,
are mentally ill, and have Alzheimer's. . .

But I am also required to listen to their broken lives,
the bleakness that has come about from losing a spouse,
a granddaughter who hung herself,
a suppurating wound on the buttocks that never heals,
the bank that has threatened to take their shacks
for inability to pay mortgage,
the son who no longer stops by to see them,
a doctor who keeps giving morphine and nothing else.

My castle walls are sturdy but there are days
when arrows chip away the mortar
and a rock from a catapult rips away a turret
and the plague seeps through slits in the windows. . .

What has happened to these people?
Have their whole lives been this horrid?
Why have their hopes come to such a standstill,
their time a bumpy downhill race to hell?
Were they ever young? Did they ever dream?
Did they not once, long ago, show potential,
eagerness to thrive? Desire that burned them with happiness?

Was there not a single happy moment they called their own. . .

PRE-DEATH CARE

Treating Colby three times in a year
and now starting the fourth go-round
I see he has not progressed in any way
and for a moment I feel I have failed.

But the moment fades and I know
I have done the best I could
for a 300+ pound man
who profits Pall Mall
each time he puffs a cigarette
and keeps a box of Hostess Cup Cakes
on the living room table
in front of the TV
he watches non-stop
even when I'm there.

"I can still do my exercises while I watch," he emphasizes,
and he's right, since he only half-circles his ankles
and half-extends his knees a maximum
of five times each
before putting a hand to his chest
and complaining of having no breath.

"That's all I can do," he wheezes
before coughing like his lungs
are ready to burst out of his toothless mouth.
Mucus dribbles down his chin; his eyes
are more bloodshot than they normally are.
He asks for a tissue and I hand him the whole box.

"You won't get any more out of me today," he states with finality.
And I know better than to even try. I get him

a glass of water from the kitchen and see
a long line of medicines arrayed on a jelly-stained counter
like a legion of mercenaries hired
to defend a kingdom that's already doomed.

He gulps down the water and sighs.

"I don't understand it," he says.
"I get dialysis every Tuesday/Thursday/Saturday,
I just started taking Oxycodone for my hip pain,
the nurse comes twice a week to change
the dressings on my open sores,
and I do the exercises you showed me way back when
every so often—at least the ones I remember.
Still, I'm not improving." He stares at me,
angry, bewildered, scared. "No, none of it's
doing any good. I don't know why they call it Health Care
when you don't get healthy again.
They should give it another name.
They should call it like it is."

A TREND WITHOUT STOP

It has gotten to the point where I do not believe
I can really help the people I drive out to treat
at their homes, the people who can't walk, or barely,
stand with stooped backs, cough and pant
at the slightest exertion beyond lifting
fork and spoon to their mouths, and are too often
lost in dementia, or returned to a state of infancy.

I force them to move their limbs a little bit,
help them shuffle with walkers or canes
across filthy floors and rugs that harbor
kingdoms of dust and bacteria.
A few I'll take outside to step on ground and gravel
and grass and see how many feet they cover
before they tell me they're done.

Then I jot down on paper or on a laptop
the results or lack of them of the twice-a-weekly
visits that might hold at bay a grave
they already are half in. But what I would really
like to jot down is how *most* of them have dug
the graves themselves, chosen lifestyles
of living off fried food and soda pop,

never exercising, plopping into their maws prescription pills
like chocolate peanuts and wondering why
life has left them with so much hurt.
And what is to blame—Ignorance? Poor genes? Tradition?
A less-than--high-school education? Or a nation
formed on consumerism where effects are unimportant. . .
Unless. . .they lead to more consumption.

KEEP IT WITHIN LIMITS

On Friday I treated Mrs. Lindy
who. . .finally after two weeks of therapy
got out of her wheelchair and walked twenty yards
with only minimal assistance. She beamed:
"Next week let's try thirty!"

Now it's Monday, and I get the news
that Mrs. Lindy had a heart attack Saturday
and died while eating dinner. She was 91.

My first patient today is also. . .ninety-one.
Inflammation on the bottom of her foot
which I treat with ultra sound, massage.

She grimaces throughout, but when I ask her
of her pain, she shakes her head:
"No pain, no gain."

I tell her, "You need to drink lots of water.
Massage breaks down toxins in the muscles,
and the toxins need to be swept from the system."

She stares at me, half-smiling.

"Okay, I'll drink my water. But does all this work mean
I can't have sex?"

Her husband's the same age, and in worse shape.
But I chuckle. "No, you don't have to cut out sex.

Just don't overdo it!"

STILL COUNTING

Only fifty years of age and already one Total Knee Reconstruction
and another due in a year or two, Kenny smokes a cigarette
while I take his blood pressure.

                              "Does this bother you, man?" he asks.
I tell him it does. He takes a long drag then mashes the butt
in an ashtray. I've been given a list of "other" problems he has
by his social worker. "Unpredictable," the woman emphasized.
"He can blow his stack; takes the slightest wrong to the worst proportions.
Attention deficit disorder. Severe mental illness. In and out of jail. . ."

Actually I've treated more dangerous characters—once in a hospital
I dressed the leg wound of a handcuffed prisoner with a brawny guard
        each side of him.
At first Kenny's not bad at all, does everything I ask, states
that he wants his knee normal so that he can get back to welding and driving
        his truck.
When he asks for a break after ambulating sixteen stairs
I sit too to fill out his progression note on a computer.
Not three words written and I hear,
"What the fuck are you doing that
for, man? You're here to treat me
not fucking waste my time while you fuck around on a computer."

I stop and look at him, the sneer on his twisted face, eyes bulging,
his bald head turning red on his five-foot Auschwitz frame.

Then I remember other details on the list: a bi-polar meth addict,
a (supposed) recovered alcoholic, born-again religious believer,
jobless from being fired too many times, homeless from refusing to pay rent,
under court order not to stalk his ex-wife or see his children. . .
A man who suddenly avoids my gaze, a patient I have to deal with,
as I now tell myself that he is not a roach I could squash with my big toe,

no, he is a human being in need, let me relax, count to ten, no, to twenty,
maybe a hundred. I am still counting when he glances at me shyly,

"God man, I'm sorry. Forgive me. Didn't mean to go off on you like that.
Just thought you were neglecting me. It. . .won't happen again.
You can put money on that. Just tell me what to do, boss.
I just want to get better. I really do. . ."

EVEN IN THIS ERA

There are homes into which I step where the first smell is death;
bodies that already put out the stench better known after burial.
Coming to treat these bodies, I cannot clench my nostrils
nor hold my breath. I smile, cheer them up, encourage their limbs
to push freely toward health. I don't ignore their pus-warm wounds,
though I do my best to make their minds ignore them.
But most of them know, a few are forgetful through dementia,
the others in denial or praying for divine miracles.
For the rarest I am the miracle. The one, who keeps the ferryman waiting
—a few days more.

CADAVER LAB

Each year state regulations require therapists
to take a seminar pertaining to their field
and this year I stand with forty others
at the local cadaver lab listening to a surgeon
speak of the spinal cord while running a gloved hand
up and down the opened spinal column
of a body on a table.

All of us put gloves on and do the same
with other bodies on tables,
touching muscles, touching bones,
feeling nerve endings and fatty tissue.

Most of us have done this before
and it's old news; a few of the younger
crowd, students maybe, look antsy,
the smell of formaldehyde
wrinkling their noses. I hear a woman
say to another: "My God, they look
just like slabs of meat."

Other speakers come and go, the hours
drone on, and soon I am more interested
in what these bodies were before
they became slabs of meat.

One old man with a mustache with one leg
amputated at the knee—did he lose it
in Korea, Vietnam, a car accident, disease?

Another man, younger, muscles like iron:
Was he murdered? Or did he succumb

36

to heat stroke playing football in summer?

An old woman, frail, tiny, hands and feet resembling claws
from arthritis—were the final days of life painful,
or did family and friends surround her with joy?

Lastly a man not old or young but nearly bald,
obese, the flesh layered with rolls of flab.
What caused him to overeat—Loneliness? Divorce?
Lack of willpower? A tendency to indulge?

There are others, and each of them lived once,
was happy, sad, with dreams and broken dreams,
and hopefully loved, with connections to people
still in the world who remember them
as more than just slabs of meat.

SOME THINGS HAVE TO BE SAID

People rarely read verse these days
and they read rhetorical verse even less,
but my job treating lonely dying people
in dilapidated rural towns and in trailers
lying hidden off dirt roads in harsh mountains
makes me realize how the urban elite, the politicos,
the computer-savvy suburbanites
live much of their lives in mental cocoons.
They live, not knowing that country-poor
are more than bad jokes and re-runs
of Hee-Haw and Petticoat Junction.
They live, unaware there are Americans

who cannot read, signing their names with X.
They live, never understanding there are more
underclass in this nation than many
third-world nations combined. They live,
and laugh, at entire populations that keep
Pat Robertson rich and pray to portraits of Jesus on the wall
—because Jesus is all there is in a miserable world.

So why write such verse. . .*for what really changes?*
These people I treat are the spine and marrow
of conservatism in America. . .but what do corporate moguls
and presidents do for them?
What have they ever done for them except
nod happily at their vote. . .

But voting is one thing, and dying another,
and I'll continue treating them as long as I can,
until someone else comes after me
to treat their children.

THE WORLD'S INDIFFERENCE

A man I treated less than a week ago has already been buried.
Dead from a massive stroke the day after I saw him,
he lies now in a Methodist graveyard in the town of Narrows
by the New River.

The day before we walked in his huge yard, stepping on oak
leaves, over acorns; he showed me his work shed,
hammers on walls, saws and rakes hanging from hooks on the rafters.
I told him he had graduated to outpatient therapy,
that he wouldn't need home care beyond this week.

He said, "I hope you come back. I like working with you.
Next time I'll how you my medals I earned in the Korean War."

But—now he's under the earth and I am still above ground.
The season inches toward winter and nowhere are there signs
acknowledging a loss greater than a scattering of leaves.
No stars have fallen from the sky, and the world is not
coming to an end. The sun shines the same as it
did when we shaded our eyes that last day.
Dusk will follow in a few hours, night after-wards.
Tomorrow, another morning. More leaves trickle down from trees,
more acorns drop unnoticed.

THREE PATIENTS SPEAKETH

1

"You hear about that man in North Carolina who robbed a bank
for $1.00 then sat down on a bench outside the same bank
and waited for the police to come and arrest him?
Said he did it just to go to prison so he could get free health care!
I swear my son's gonna do the same thing one of these days.
He ain't had work in over two years and nobody around here's hiring.
He's suffered from ulcers for God knows how long
and now our doctor's diagnosed him with diabetes.
Damn it, he's only 43. I was still kicking ass at that age.
Jesus, I don't have the money to help him. Or the health.
And don't get me started about the goddamned government
—those sons of bitches line their own pockets and no one else's. . .
It does seem awful strange that jailbirds and politicians
receive free medical assistance while the rest of us have to mortgage
      our homes
just so the pharmacy can fill our daily prescription of pills."

2

"This therapy has really helped me—I don't know why I can't continue.
You say it's because of medicare guidelines, something about
treatments having to be skilled or else they won't pay.
But it's not my fault that I'm bed-bound, that I can't move my legs
and need oxygen 24/7. You moving them for me is good
for my circulation, good for my muscles. Can't you tell them that?
Can't you tell them the car accident I had twelve years ago
crushed my lower vertebrae and left me so that a caretaker
has to wipe my rear end and remove the soiled sheets of my bed
several times a day. Can't you tell them that my mind is still clear
and that I don't want to die just yet. I still have a lot to do,
I want to play with my grandchildren, I want to feel the river-wind
after a rain and eat the first ear of corn picked from our garden.

Don't things like that count? Doesn't anything count anymore. . ."

3

"Listen, I realize you mean well. I realize you're trying to get me
to walk again, to step outside this Old Folks Home, but what's the point?
My daughter put me here because she herself couldn't
care for me. . .or *wouldn't*. And everyone with half a brain knows
this place is just a junkyard for beaten-down cars.
No, I don't have much longer, and frankly it doesn't matter.
It doesn't matter at all. I've lived my life—some of it good,
some bad, most of it just plain hard work with a little reward here and there.
So son, don't waste your time. You got other patients to tend to.
Patients more likely to do the exercises you want them to do.
I'd rather be left alone. All of us die only once,
so at least let me die the way I choose to die.
It's not everyone that gets that choice."

WINTER OF NO SUMMER

Six months ago she walked up two steps at a time
and returned to planting tomatoes like she had done
before her first fall. Now she has fallen a second time,
fractured her pelvis, and sits slumped in a wheelchair
terrified not only to attempt to walk, but to stand
even for ten seconds on her own without clawing my arms
and pleading, "Please don't let me fall! I don't want to fall again!"

And though I tell her I'll never let her fall—
and that if she ever wants to walk freely
without someone bracing her shoulders and hips
then she needs to start this moment or else
her muscles will atrophy and it will be too late
—she stares at me wildly and shakes her head.

"You just don't understand. Once you've fallen like I have
you're never the same. My legs won't work
and my mind can't get them to work.
So please. . .don't make me try something I can't do.
I'd rather die than go through the agony of lying
five hours alone on the ground. You must understand that.
I'd rather die. . ."
              But I am still young, and I don't understand.
I don't know what it's like to lie on the grass
not being able to get up. Screaming in pain for help,
wondering why none of the neighbors, the mailman, a child on a tricycle,
hears.

DEMOCRACY OR CORPOCRACY

It was inevitable the question would come up:
"What do *you* think of our health care system?"

The person who asks: a sixty year old man
with Multiple Sclerosis, wheelchair-bound, fallen
five times in the last month, despite full
Hospice care and physical and occupational therapy
three sessions a week, each. He can't bathe himself,
has trouble holding a fork or spoon, slurs his words,
wears pampers, and forgets half the things you tell him.

But his question is clear, and how can I answer. . .

It works for some; for others it works barely;
for some it doesn't work at all. The figures are frightening:
40 to 60 million Americans without health care benefits.
Millions more paying the bulk of their paychecks
with a few cents leftover for food. But I don't
inform him of these facts. Neither do I say
that corporations hold the system like a boa constrictor
and what always comes first to them
is not individual care, but the numbers of patients,
the numbers of profits, the numbers of hours
medical staff can be (il)legally overworked
without compensation.

No, I just look at him and shrug. Why relay the news
that in ten days his insurance will run out
and we won't be able to treat him.
                              "Probably best
I don't say anything either way," I suggest.
"You'd only get an opinion. . .but I might lose my job."

FIRST PATIENT OF THE DAY

There comes a time when no good is found
turning anguish into art. Like today
when I treat an eighty year old
with Alzheimer's
who forgets two minutes after I tell him my name
and occupation
why I have come to see him.

And his wife who keeps asking me
whether he'll be well again
when she isn't well herself
being mostly deaf
never hearing what I say
even after half-screaming
two inches from her ear.

And the fat, dwarf-like son
with the John Adams hairstyle
who has never left home
and now at fifty-seven
sits in a chair in the living room
all day
watching TV
and berating his parents
for being imbeciles
either through words of disgust
or shaking his fists at them
while probably contemplating
murder.

There comes a time when no good is found
turning anguish into art, for it won't

change a damned thing,
but I do it anyway,
mainly
to keep my own
sanity.

THE WARS WE NEVER HEAR ABOUT

Nora'll never receive a medal for raising eight children
(often without a husband or boyfriend),
feeding them, clothing them, seeing seven survive to adulthood,
the other one. . .die from leukemia. She won't get a call
from the president for battling through her own cancer
off-and-on for five years, parts of them confined to a wheelchair,
nor will her governor acknowledge that after going
to an outpatient clinic for four months
she's now able to walk half a mile without fainting.

There'll won't be a plaque on the wall of congress commemorating Ron
for 27 years of working construction and building interstate highways
since he was seventeen, not a week of vacation in his life
unless he was laid off or had trouble finding a road that needed fixing,
with hardly a day of sick leave since he was the only breadwinner
    of the family.
He won't even receive a letter from the mayor for regaining
full range of motion after having his rotator cuff repaired.

No movie will ever be made of Martin who lost a leg at the hip
when he fell under the blades of a tractor a day
before his high school graduation. No film crew
to show footage of his beet-red face and the grunts
that empty from his lungs like bellows when he pushes
a hundred-plus pounds on the leg press machine
twenty times without stop.

And Tammy has yet to be interviewed by CNN
for improving her posture and the ability to sleep at night
with decreased pain. Having scoliosis detected
when she was three, she lived a decade with back discomfort
that left her disfigured and unable to go to school

46

or participate in church league soft ball. But thrice-a-week aquatic therapy
and daily stretching techniques allow her
to step with barely a limp and swing a bat
with no sign of a crooked torso.

WEAK BREAKWATERS

It's been three months since I last treated him
so the phone call this afternoon from his wife
in a voice straining caught me unaware:
"Just wanted to tell you that Tucker died
this past Friday. And wanted to thank you
for all you did. He really liked you, and,
he *did* get better. Was able to walk around
the house with barely any pain, and even
sometimes around the yard. And he never
fell a single time since getting therapy.
He was grateful for your help. I'm grateful.
Thank you. He passed away just like he wanted to:
at home. That's all he wanted; all the family
wanted. Thank you again, and good luck
with your job. Bye now. . ."
                              She hung up
so fast I couldn't even ask how, not that it
matters. Death is final. Words and condolences
weak breakwaters against fate.

Though once, I thought otherwise. . .

As a child watching Wiley Coyote
continually blow himself to smithereens
seeking to detonate the Road Runner, but always
returning sound and whole of body,
I think somewhere in the brain
I perceived mortality as a game of King of the Hill
where the loser never ceased to march the slope.

Even when my grandparents left one by one
I believed at most they'd be gone a few days,

48

before seeing them again smiling and laughing
at Sunday dinner. Either I was too young,
or the adult-world as usual became tight-lipped
about all that is real, and gave me a cupcake
and a toy and sat me in front of the TV
to watch more cartoons. . .
                              But even the best
insulation doesn't last. I know Tucker
won't come back. Nor any other patients
I treated who have since died.
Neither my Father or a girl I dated whose spine
was crushed by a tractor-trailer.

They don't come back, and they don't tell you
where they've gone. The slope they've fallen down
is an inescapable void—too massive to not notice,
but as small and distant as a pinprick in a dark sea.
I can't lift up the phone and ask them how they are.
I can't offer them any therapy that will
make them walk the hill again.

VICTIMS NO LESS

For Patty

I had never spoken to his wife Becca
except on the phone when I called
to set up an appointment or to ask
for details about the disease and paralysis
that he couldn't remember
or purposely wanted to forget.

But today an aide gives him a bath while I wait
in the living room, and Becca, who must have
hoped for such an occasion says,
"I'm sure you see a lot of cases like this. . ."

When I nod she breaks out in tears, putting
a hand over her eyes, moaning, "I'm sorry.
I'm sorry. I'm sorry. I wanted to tell you
something but I know you've got
more important things on your mind. . ."

Instinctively I realize her tears are because of Len.
Unfortunately I *have* seen such cases, too many:
A man of 38 who suddenly starts getting seizures
baffling first the family, then the doctors,
who can no longer drive or fit drain pipes
into the ground because it is too dangerous
and a hazard for his health and the wellbeing
of his colleagues. Gone with his ability
to walk or even stand are salary and benefits;
the wheelchair he uses is bought second-hand.

I say, "We're going to do what we can for him.

There might. . .*Yes, there might be a chance*
we can progress him to crutches and even a cane.
But, he will have to help us out.
He can't expect to improve if he doesn't
want to do the exercises and gives up
before at least trying."

A few tissues grabbed to absorb the sniffling,
Becca inhales and exhales before speaking.
"That's the problem," she states, "he's already
given up. It's been a year now since he first fell
and cut open his head, and ever after
he cusses me whenever I plead with him to try,
try, try, you gotta try, Len. Not only for yourself,
but for me, and the kids. . ."
                              A pause.
I don't fill it with words. She continues.
"You said you know other cases. Well, my question is:
How do families in these situations respond?
I want to live too! I don't want to go through the next ten years
watching him wither away, no longer able to speak,
or eat without tubes, putting pampers on him
and feeling the misery in his eyes
as he envies my legs that take me places,
and silently—and sometimes *loudly*—accuses me
for going on while he lapses into apathy.
I don't want to spend the good years of my life
bearing guilt for an affliction I never caused.
His friends and parents say I'm selfish
to carry these thoughts, but they're not the ones
who have to take the kids to an amusement park alone,
to the baseball games and ballet, to make certain
they get on the school-bus safely
and get off safely, they don't have to come home
worn out from work but still needing
to cook dinner, clean dishes, wash clothes,
put everyone to bed. Do you know Len and I
used to go to the movies once a week;

51

we haven't gone in six months. He's either
too embarrassed about being in a wheelchair
or worried 'bout peeing his pants.
I went to two films with a girlfriend
but it's just not the same. And one of the times
afterwards Len alleged I was out having an affair.
Dear Lord, such a thing's never crossed my mind!"

I am speechless for awhile. My job is to treat
her husband's physical ailments: decreased mobility,
decreased strength, lack of range of motion.
I tell her we can arrange a social worker
to come by to help with domestic needs,
but she says they have a social worker
and that nothing's changed.
                                          "I shouldn't have said
what I did," she adds quickly, as I lock eyes with her,
knowing she craves a hug—though protocol
and professionalism won't allow it.

Fresh tears fall and she opens her mouth,

only to close it. The aide wheels Len into the room
with the smell of bath soap and shampoo.
He squints his eyes at me; he squints at his wife.

"You been here long?" he asks me suspiciously.

"No," I answer. "I just got here a few minutes ago."

MOST PATIENTS TALK ABOUT THE WEATHER

There are breaks between gait training
and teetering on a balance board
when Letta catches her breath, saying,
This reminds me of bad times. Then quickly:
No, no, no,—not you! I mean the exercises. . .
No, that's not right either, I love exercising.
I wouldn't be 89 now if I hadn't swum
and walked every day and learned yoga.
It's just. . .nearly losing my balance like that
makes me remember grabbing hold of loose bricks
when the world was coming to an end.

And when I look perplexed: *Of course it was*
long before you were born. Long before.
The Americans by day, the British by night.
What an awful time that was! I was a only a young woman.
It seems I spent half my youth living in bomb shelters.
Dodging falling ruins. Picking my way through rubble.
We lost our apartment—the entire building flattened!
Other buildings beside it were half-destroyed,
the walls smashed, revealing rooms with charred sofas,
leaky bathtubs suspended by a few drainage pipes in the air,
scattered shoes and cabinets, mangled pianos.
Whole streets were like that! Whole sections of Berlin.
It was then I knew Hitler was evil.
Oh, we all thought in the beginning: What a beautiful man!
*We **believed** in what he told us. . .*
He had built us back up from scratch after the Depression.
Then right before the invasion of Poland
my father pounded his fist on the table one night at dinner:

That man's going to get us into war!
Then everything only got worse. . .
The best luck I had was leaving the city before the Russians came;
my closest girlfriend stayed and was raped by 27 of them.
Me—I met an American officer who brought me over here.. .

Oh, Brian, some things we shouldn't think again.
Alright, what exercise next?

For a few moments I'm too speechless to tell her.

"Okay. . .let's try standing on one foot."

THE 26TH MISSION

I couldn't help asking Bill about his past
after noticing the baseball hat he always wears
with the 15th Air Force insignia
and all the paintings, photos, and plastic models
of B-24 Liberators decking his walls and desks.
When he huffs and puffs after finishing
20 repetitions of half-squats he asks for a rest
and I say:

"So how did you become a bomber pilot?"

He shrugs. "The boys up top wanted me to fly
a Mustang, but I put my foot down—as much
as you're ever able to in the military.
I never wanted to be a fighter pilot.
Didn't want to see the men I had to kill."

He pauses. "Of course, I'm sure I killed people.
Though it wasn't the intent. Our goal
was always to hit railroad depots and supply trains,
munitions factories, ball-bearing plants,
anything of war-making potential.
I was based in Italy. Usually we flew up to Germany:
Dusseldorf, Dresden, Berlin, sometimes Austria,
the Ploesti oil fields in Romania,
a few raids targeting bridges in Yugoslavia,
and once we even took out an armaments plant in Poland."

He pauses again. "Yes, I'm sure some people died.
When you fly 25 missions (and very few bombing crews
even made half that many runs) you drop a lot of bombs.
Luckily, I only lost one man the whole time.

One of the tail gunners didn't make it.
Several others got wounded. A co-pilot
got his ankle shattered by a bullet.
That was a rough ride home.
On the same mission a bullet flew right by my head.
But you had to keep flying. Had to return to base.
On another occasion we barely reached the target area
when the plane in front of us was mangled by flak
and broke in pieces. Disintegrated before our eyes. . .
We saw all of the men parachute out—all except the pilot.
Either he couldn't scramble out in time
or he was dead already. Strangely, I never thought
about losing my own life; when you're 21
you're God's gift to the world and the hell
with anyone who tells you differently.
But the missions became easier towards the end.
By the winter and spring of '45 the Germans
had lost too many good pilots, too many planes.
All the new pilots were inexperienced, underage.
Our own fighters usually blew them out of the sky."

He eyes me sternly, his 90 year old vision still strong.

"I want to tell you," he states calmly, "in no way
did I like. . .war. Most of it's fear and drudgery. Boredom.
Being away from home. Eating the same rations
day in, day out. Returning to base after flying
nearly twenty hours in sub-arctic temperatures
and finding empty bunks—that would never again
be used by friends you knew. The same friends
you'd eaten dinner and played cards with the night before."

He makes a noise between a sigh and a growl.

"You just want to get it over with," he adds emphatically.
"You just want to win and go home.
I can't speak for everyone. I knew daredevil pilots
who flew planes like Babe Ruth hitting home runs,

56

trouncing the enemy without a bit of remorse.
That wasn't me. Do your job. Fulfill the quota.
End the war. Fly back stateside.
And that's what I did. . ."

He is quiet with a far-off look. I say:

"Bill, if you want to, we can call it a session.
I think I wore you out today with the new exercises."

Again he stares at me sternly.

"Hell, son, I'm no quitter. You just tell me what to do,
and I'll do it!"

HUMPTY DUMPTY

Today a patient tries to engage me in a political conversation
while I check his pulse and blood pressure and later his temperature
which are all borderline dangerous.
Says he's tired of the "shit" we have now in office
and doesn't appreciate the government putting a noose around everything
in the whole "goddamned" country.

He stops with the yapping for a while when trying to stand
with his eyes closed and when using his cane to maneuver
down four steps from his patio to a grassy back yard
that needs mowing.
                    "Can't get good help these days," he grouses,
stepping cautiously through the dandelions and weeds.
"The youngsters are just too lazy and the lawn services
charge too much. I ain't got money to waste paying jackasses
who never do the job right anyway. That's why I need
to feel better so I can get this yard looking halfway decent again."

Then after five shaky push ups on a wall and barely able to breathe
he returns to politics: "If I have to pay any more taxes to those bastards
in Washington with their grandiose dreams and liberal-faggot ideas
I might just take my gun up there and shoot someone!"

Then seeing me startled: "Nah! I don't really mean that.
I ain't that desperate. But I know people who are.
You can't stick good people's noses in shit forever
without them one day throwing it right back at you,
and worse. You just wait and see. There's a lot of grumbling
in this country of ours, and there's gonna be hell to pay
if changes aren't made—the type of *changes* we want!"

The words are nearly out of my mouth to tell him
(though professional tact keeps me mum and nodding)
that he should forget about the carnival up north
and instead concentrate on making sure he can get
to the bathroom without falling. Just last week he slid
on a wet towel and fell in the tub. Lucky he only scraped
his wrist and bruised a shoulder. If he had broken
his pelvis or a hip, or cracked his skull. . .then not even
God could have put him back in complete order,
let alone a senator or president of his choice.

THE AGE OF COMMUNICATION

I have been to the house a half a dozen times
but when I ring the doorbell an old woman
peers through the eye-hole and says,
"We're not letting you in! You're an escaped criminal!"

"Mrs. Bagley, it's me, Brian. I've been treating
your husband Gerald for the past three weeks.
Don't you remember?"
                           Then the door opens, a crack,
a little more, a beady eye raking me, then two eyes,
a frightened face. "We thought you were the fugitive."
She lets me in. "A convict's broken out of the local jail.
There's been a shooting. We heard it on the news.
Just a mile or so down the road. Didn't you know?"

Three treatments done and thirty minutes from the last one
I have heard nothing but the groans from a cancer patient
and the aches from a woman with every known ailment
since time began, and the roll of tires and a message
from the office stating that Mr. Feldrum had canceled
his 1:30 appointment due to constipation. But no word
of any convict.
                           "Mother, leave the man alone!" a voice
screeches from the living room. The couple's only son,
a man nearly seventy who's never left home
glares at the woman; smiles at me. "My father's
ready for therapy."
                           I try to smile back. His sire
Gerald lies asleep on a recliner, not rising
even when I greet him and take his blood pressure.
Though it's the same every time. He wakes occasionally
to ask if I'm the gas-man, then when I tell him to do a few exercises,

60

he does them—then asks me again if I'm the gas-man.

"Why does the gas-man want me to exercise?" he says to his wife.
But she's hard of hearing, and when she doesn't answer
he falls asleep again. Just then the back-door opens
and Mrs. Bagley screams. "Jordy, don't go out there! You'll be killed!"

"Mother. . .I am sixty-five years old! You can't tell me
what I can or can't do. Just shut up!"

He goes out, gazes at the woods to the west
where a fat water tower sits quietly on a hill.
He returns, slams the door. "There's nothing to be afraid of, Mother.
So not another peep about fugitives on the loose."

"Oh Jordy, you shouldn't treat your mother like this. . ."

"Shut up!"

He's about to say more when Gerald opens his eyes,
stares at me, puzzled. "What's the gas-man doing here?
"We don't owe any money do we?"

LESSON OF THE DAY

Rarely is Dobson well enough after chemotherapy
—even two or three days after—to perform more than moving
his feet up and down and circling his ankles
clockwise and counter-clockwise. The infrared unit
strapped to his calves and thighs he doesn't mind
for it gives about the only sensation he feels below the knees.

The victim of a stroke and now succumbing to pancreatic cancer
he tells me in a low voice how he misses cigars,
"—just a smoke here and there would do me wonders.
But they won't let me. My wife's in cahoots with the doctor
and my daughter berates me: 'Daddy, you know that's
what caused this mess in the first place.' But they don't understand,
it don't matter anymore. I know I'm done for. I know it.
So what could puffing on one cigar do that it's not already done. . ."

I have no ready answer. In these situations there is no answer.
A person dying is a person dying and for the living, the surviving
people of the world to explain factual correctness to one
craving one last moment of addiction before entering the grave
sounds like a hangman withholding the final wish.

Restricted by protocol I nod with wordless sympathy.
I'm only here to offer a little pain management, a few techniques
to help with blood circulation, standing stability, stepping strategies
to get him from his bed to the toilet and back without stumbling
or tripping on the rug. He tolerates these few options
for his world is a bed and walking several minutes a day
and nothing more. Or at least I thought so. . .

"Man, I could move like the wind once upon a time," he echoes
as though reading my thoughts. "I built my own house.

I built many of the houses in this neck of the woods.
You ever been here before. . .I mean to **Wild Banks**?"

I tell him I've never treated anyone in this town
without a post office, or restaurant, or even a single store.
Never even heard of it before weaving through windy roads
and up and down hills and past silos and farmlands
scanning my atlas to find it not far from the New River.

"A lot of folks don't know about Wild Banks," he says, closing his eyes.
"It's the only Black community in the entire area.
The same families have lived here since the end of the Civil War."

I tell him I had no idea.

"Yes siree, this community goes back a long ways.
Our people were all slaves working the local river plantations.
Then after the war, after freedom, the plantation owners
said they still needed us to tend the crops.
We were free, but we didn't have anywhere to go.
We needed them as much as they needed us.
So they got together and picked this spot of land
and gave it to us, gave us enough land to farm on our own,
raise pigs and chickens, and a few of us even got rich
and bought horses and wagons, to sell apples and corn in town."

History was my major in college but mostly I only remember
the dates of far-off wars and names of kings who lost their heads.
But here is a man before me with a history unrecorded
in annals or books or even regional almanacs.
I tell him he knows more about his history than I know of my own.

"Well, we all have a history," he concludes, "for better or worse.
I wouldn't trade mine with nobody's. In Wild Banks you can leave
your doors unlocked at night, and people always call to tell you
your car windows are down when it rains. Usually they won't even
bother calling but will go out and close them for you.
And they always bring food by when you're sick. . ."

He pauses. Opens his eyes. Looks at me pointedly.

"Folks have been doing that a *lot* for me lately.
I'm just sad I won't be able to repay them."

NO WALLS HIGH ENOUGH

Treating the lonely and dying does get to me.
I'd be lying if I said otherwise.
The days when the only patients I treat
are ones whose minds have solidified to cement,
whose bodies are no longer bodies
but bones and appendages no fuel or magic potion can lift.

It bothers me to see such helplessness beyond help.
The knowledge I take home after work remembering
Mrs. Retty who lies comatose and demented,
frequently weeping or yelling out names
while her caregiver tells me not to worry about it,
"She's like this every day."

It hurts in ways I can't explain to family or friends,
knowing Harry will wear diapers the rest of his life
and have his ass wiped by a hospice worker
before being tucked into bed with towels
wrapped under his chin to catch the drool.

It leaves me wondering seriously why I do this job
knowing I can do so little for Douglas
whose one glory out of each day
is the spoon-fed applesauce his house-sitter
gives him as a reward for not peeing in his wheelchair.

It leaves me wondering as well which is worse. . .
treating Mr. Kord who has stopped listening to his children,
stopped listening to me, stopped eating, spits his medicine out at the nurse
and refuses to exercise, refuses to quit smoking and drinking,
and won't open the door to the cleaning lady.
"Just leave me the hell alone! All of you!

I'm going to croak soon anyway."

Or hoping that Sallie Rose will understand her limited ability
and not expect to drive every other weekend to her sister in Richmond
like she has for nearly two decades. "But I only had three crashes. . .
And no one got injured. Well, except for me. Though I don't
recall blacking out. And it's not because I'm weak!
I still go up and down my stairs every so often.
I'm not going to be homebound forever—I'll tell you that much!
It's all because of the winter. Once summer comes this arthritis
won't be as bad. I'll perk up again. You'll see.
And those new pills the doc's giving me are gonna
cure my heartburn and dizziness. You'll see."

I do see. Though there are times I'd rather not see anything
but four sturdy walls without windows
containing a quiet world of no cancer cells or fractured hips,
a world without the smell of shit-stained gowns
and the pleas of people always asking me,
"Do you think my Mom will one day be able to walk?
Do you think she'll be sturdy enough to cook in her own kitchen?
Or do we need to. . .need to find another place. . .for her. . . to live?"

POSTER BOY

Zeb is one of those patients I could work with a million years
and never grow tired of seeing. Eighty-eight turnings
around the sun and he still gets up every morning
and walks around his yard, putting bird seed in feeders
and watching squirrels gather acorns.
                                        "It was only the one time
I fell," he says, grinning. "And that's because I tripped over
a damned branch. Even a kid can do that! I got right back up, too.
Only bruised my hip, and my back was sore a couple of weeks.
But nothing else! Then my son who's never worried
about me before thinks I need to move into an Old Folks Home.
Hell, my wife's been dead since '91 and I've lived here on my own
alone, still driving, still painting the barn every summer,
still planting corn and hoeing the good earth."

Trim to a point that's unusual for a man his age
he wipes sweat from his forehead after doing the squats
I ask him to do to build leg strength. "I've been doing squats
my whole life. I've been working my whole life."

"Zeb, you're one of the healthiest persons I've treated," I tell him.
'We could make a poster of you to show how fit the elderly
could all be if they took care of themselves."

He laughs. "Well, there really ain't nothing to it.
I just don't let nothing worry me. And I'll be damned
if I stay cooped up inside from dawn till dusk.
I need to get out and cut the grass, trim the hollies,
pick apples, pull weeds from the tomato patch.
I grew up on a farm in Tazewell County,
and my daddy was the same. Working from before the sun rose,
never complaining, doing what had to be done.

That's how life's supposed to be! Enjoy your work
and the rest will take care of itself.
I ain't got time for people that watch TV all day.
If the Good Lord had wanted us to do that—
he'd have made the damned things in the first place.
Now. . .you want me to do more squats or hop on one leg?"

YOU PICK: EVOLUTION OR MADE IN THE IMAGE OF GOD

My second day in Home Health with orientation enough
just to acquaint me with the local terrain
I head to Barren Springs, near Wythe County, Virginia.
When my supervisor said it's a long drive into the middle of nowhere
I thought she was partly joking, but this place is beyond that.
A little road that's not even on the map
partly gravel, partly pot-holes
and nowhere to turn in case I'm going the wrong way.

Why did I take this job, I half-scream to myself,
45 minutes into the journey and still counting
until I finally find the address, a rusty mailbox next to a dead tree.
I slowly creep up the dirt driveway, spotting
a wheel-less Chevy Impala propped on cinder-blocks,
next to it an old pick-up with four flat tires
and a tractor that looks like the first one ever made.

I park the car near a cage where a pit bull pops up from the ground, barking.
It leaps at the chained links as I scout the cage hoping
there's no hole. Sighing, I get my medical bags and walk to the front door
of a trailer that looks like a cross between a log cabin splotched with mold
and a larger-than-normal outhouse.
I knock.

Voices behind the door. It opens. A woman smiling with one tooth.

"Can I help you, sir?"

"I'm here to see Ralph Menkins for physical therapy," I say.

"Oh. . .that's our Dad." She turns. "Daddy, the therapist man is here."

She waves a hand and I enter. Another toothless woman is sitting
holding a beer, watching *As the World Turns.* She smiles, blushing.

"Normally we don't start this early."

Four empty bottles sit on a table near her chair.
The other woman lifts a half-filled bottle from the table
and takes a swig. "That's my sister, Tamra"—she points
to the sitting woman—"and you can call me Tabby."

Tamra pulls out a cigarette and lights it.

"I hope you don't mind us smoking.
We'll try not to blow it in your direction.
Now Daddy, you get up out of that sofa and sit up.
This man's here to treat you."

Ralph, who's 78 according to the Evaluation document
opens his eyes and groans as if he's been slugged.

"What'd you say, Tamra?"

"She said the therapist needs to treat you!'
Tabby shakes her head, takes a cigarette from her sister, lights it.

"Who?" The old man rolls up and groans again.

Tabby winks at me. "He can be ornery at times,
so don't mind him a bit. The last therapist to see him
was a pretty young girl—not to say that you're not pretty!—
but I think he took a likin' to her.
But she only came out the one time.
Now that I think of it, we seem to have a new therapist every week.
Must have gone through three or four in the last month.
I don't know why. Daddy ain't that hard to work with."

The old man has scrunched up his eyes and is staring at me.

"So. . .you're the therapist? What happened to that little girl
that was coming. . ."

"I'm not sure," I say. "They never told me at the office.
They just put you on my schedule and sent me out to see you.
Are you doing okay?"

"I reckon I am. I'm still alive, aren't I.
And I don't really need no therapy.
It's these two young uns here
that keep saying I need therapy."

"Daddy, now you behave." Tamra blows a puff of smoke at me
that burns my nostrils. "You know you had that fall
in the backyard and nearly broke your spine.
This man's here to help you. So let him help you!"

Ralph grumbles as I unscroll the blood pressure cuff
and am about to circle it around his arm
when I see his skin is crusted with a brown
scab-like appearance.

"Ralph—is that a bruise on your arm?" I ask, never having
seen such massive discoloration covering one spot.

"No, sonny, that ain't no bruise. That's just tobacco spit.
Whenever I fall asleep it dribbles out of my mouth
and stains my clothes and arms. But it won't bother you."

Knowing I have sanitary wipes in my bag I proceed,
trying my best not to gag. I take all his vitals
and they are surprisingly good. I get him to perform
a few exercises sitting, then standing,
before he tells me he needs a break.
Then bending over he picks up a pickle jar the size of a bucket,
three quarters full of a swirling black paste.

"This thing's getting heavy," he states, loosing
a wad of spit into the center of the dark muck.
"I'm gonna dump this thing in the sink then I'll be right back."

Tabby follows him into the kitchen. "Daddy,
I'm gonna make some lunch. You want some too?"

"Hell yeah!" I hear him exclaim as the sound of gushing liquid
pours down a drain.

He returns.

"Sonny, I've had about all the exercise I can tolerate today.
Lifting that jar just about did me in."

There's nothing I can do but nod as Ralph plops
into the sofa again and Tabby brings in
a bologna on white, two Twinkies and a Bud Lite.

"When you coming again?" she asks, with a one-toothed grin.

"I'll. . .have to check with the office," I say.
"It—could be they put Ralph on my schedule by mistake."

"They must be putting him on everyone's schedule by mistake."
She continues to grin. "Would you like a beer before you go?"

"No, I'm fine," I say. "I really am, I'm fine."
Then turn to the car. And go.

TO LISTEN IS TO LEARN

I had been warned by a nurse who had attended Mrs. Gleedy,
"Not only will she talk non-stop from the time you arrive
till the time you leave, but she complains about everything
including the president, her doctors, and even God.
So talk as little as possible or you'll never get out of there."

Well, complaining's old as the human race, and no subject
is taboo. So I set up the ultra sound unit, time it ten minutes,
squeeze the gel around her right knee, run the soundhead
smoothly over the swelling, all the while listening to her voice
that's like a bagpipe out of tune: "Do you know my son,
that lazy good-for-nothing (and I'd say worse
but I'm afraid it might offend you), won't even offer
to mow my lawn anymore. And I even said I'd pay him!
Just a few weeks ago I asked him to take me to the voting booth
and he never even showed up, and damn if he ever answers
his phone. Not that the voting really mattered.
Those candidates promise you the world then when they become
senators they sit on their ass. . .their *rear ends* in Washington
and forget all about the state they even came from.
Who needs them! They're almost as bad as my doctors.
Honey, do you know I've gone through more than a dozen doctors
in the past five years! Five years! And not one of the bunch
has been able to tell me why my knee aches so much.
They all say it's arthritis and old age, but they probably say
the same to everyone. And I never have figured out why
my back hurts all the time. And no, don't say it's because
my bed's too lumpy, or that I lie on the sofa half the day.
A person my age is entitled to taking it easy,
and I don't aim to do any differently. I worked
fixing school lunches for nearly thirty years
so I deserve a little rest. But all those doctors ever do
is give me more pills: pills, pills, pills. My God,

73

I hate the lot of them. And even the Lord's not being
good to me. I pray, who knows how many times a day
and all I get is more pain. All I want is to feel better.
To be able to wake every morning without a knife
stabbing me from the middle of my back down to my knee.
Other folks pray for a house at the beach and they get it.
Damn the lot of them! Those people don't know what pain's like.
My neighbor thinks I'm being too harsh in my thoughts
so I finally gave her a piece of my mind. Haven't spoken
to her since, and that was months ago. Well, I wasn't
put on earth to please her. I'll be damned if—"

I glance at the timer: 2 minutes to go. Continue
to move the soundhead. Then I'll wipe the knee clean
and pack up the machine. A few exercises
and balancing techniques afterward, a few transfers,
an assessment for functional mobility. I notice
the room is quiet. Her eyes are glaring.

"Honey, I don't think you heard what I just said!"

"I'm sorry, I was checking the machine."

"Well, that's the problem with the world today,
we rely too much on machines. Did I tell you
about the time I went to get my eyes looked at
and they had me stare into this contraption
that looked like something from outer space.
My God, I got so dizzy I thought I was going to die.
Then they tried to get me to buy some fancy new glasses.
And would you believe how much they cost?
I could've bought groceries for four months
for the price of those damned glasses.
And groceries ain't cheap either these days.
Just this last week I planned to buy some peaches
to make a cobbler and you know how much
they were selling for? Honey. . .are you still listening to me?
Honey. . ."

NOT EVEN HIPPOCRATES

Mel does everything I ask of him, though always afterward
his chest heaves like he's just outraced a cheetah.
Today he huffs, "Son, you might have to go a little easier on me
with the exercises. And I don't want to walk out in the grass today.
I'm almost ninety and darned lucky to have made it this far."

I tell him he's healthier than most people his age
but he shakes his head. "No, I'm not. I'm just lucky."
And when I don't respond he takes off his glasses, rubs his eyes.
"What I mean is, all my friends who worked with me
in the mines have long passed on. All the years
they breathed in the coal dust—**BLACKENED THEIR LUNGS!**
I know it did the same to me—but I'm still here."

I'm more amazed than he is. "How long did you work in the mines?"

"Practically all my life. Seems that way. My daddy
left the family one day and never came back.
So me being the oldest, I had to earn what I could for my Momma.
There were eight of us children and rarely did we have food
enough for all of us, or shoes, and the house-rent
each month took nearly everything we had."

"What about school? How'd you manage school with all the work?"

Shaking his head again he brands me with his eyes a fool.

"I never went to school. Never read no books,
heck I never even learned to write. You've seen that for yourself
each time you come here and I have to sign your computer
with a check mark. Weren't no time, and I'm not even sure
I'd have gone anyway. Some of my sisters went,

and a few of my brothers, though all the boys
ended up in the mine with me except for one of them.
He was only nine and got hit by a car while crossing a road."

He pauses a moment. "The others are all gone now too.
Two of my sisters are still alive, but I ain't seen them
for goodness knows how many years. Life goes by quickly.
All my friends and family have left."

His words touch me and he senses it. "Yes, life goes quickly,"
he states again, looking me in the eye. "You'd better live
while you still have lungs in you. All those boys
who came out of the mines every evening, smiling
when the work-day was done. Well, they didn't smile that long.
Unless they're smiling in heaven right now." He stops again.
"And I'm not so sure of that. What do you think?
Are these exercises I'm doing gonna bring me closer to my loved ones?"

I keep quiet. Not even Hippocrates could fully answer such a question.
And no one else I know of can either.

NO OTHER FACT MATTERS

We all of us have our church, our wine, our easel, our ocean
to stare at when the world is suddenly wrong
and words of comfort lack power or peace,
and the voices of the dead speak stronger
and we wonder why we live, still,
when others around us have gone to a place
where clarity is not a byword
and faith is always undefined.

For me, I come to a tiny waterfall
part of a stream leading to a greater river
to find in the water running over gray granite
the reason why a man I treated in recent weeks
has died. A victim of fractured vertebrae
and a torn achilles he had just learned again
to walk, with a cane, indoors and outdoors
on gravel and grass and up and down stairs
and the last I saw of him he smiled, saying,
"I'm getting better each time I see you."

The dark current rushes by me, rushes by weeds and oaks
and wind-carved stones not explaining anything
I want explained. Is it too much to ask why death
too often gives us no warning? A sun shining,
then blocked by clouds, never to shine again.
Is it nihilistic to wonder if there are things we are not meant to know,
questions not meant to be answered? Or is there reason
for everything, a fate meted out beyond reasoning?

The falls burples with unperturbed quiet.
Should I seek another spot for understanding. . .
I throw a pebble in the water. Watch circles widen, then vanish.

I throw another. The same occurs. I throw a third.
What difference would there be if I threw forever?
An accumulation of pebbles at the bottom of the stream?
A temporary obstruction to the flow of water? What else?
The simple summary: the man I treated is gone.

A LIFE IN A DAY

Eighty-three and limber enough to teach yoga
Marge has only the occasional neck and gluteal pain
from sitting too long alone in her one bedroom
ground floor apartment with a gray cat named Chester.
She watches TV because, "I never had a TV until I got older.
I'm making up for it now. I was married when I was 15,
back then you were an old maid if you didn't have a husband
by 21. Heck, I already had three children before that age.
My first husband ran off after the second baby
and I heard later he joined the Marines, went to Korea,
and never came back. With my second husband
I had three more children. One of them died, a boy.
And one of my grandsons died too a few years ago,
in his sleep, heart attack. Only thirty-two.
Good Lord, life is like a lightning streak. . .then it's gone.
I tell my youngest granddaughter—'Now honey,
don't you dare get married until you are at least forty.
You got to live a little, go to school, earn some money,
meet the boys when you're ready for them.'
Though I don't know how much she'll listen.
She's a freshman in high school and they're already knocking
down the door. I buried my second man before
I was even seventy. He had ten years on me
and couldn't walk or talk in the end after two strokes.
I gave up my job cleaning rooms at the hospital
which I'd done fourteen years, just to take care of him.
But I doubt he even knew it was me; I could have been
the neighbor or a paid caregiver to wipe the drool
that dripped all the time from his mouth
(and wiped other things as well!)
for by then he didn't even know who *he* was.
I never want to get like that. I told my children,

if I ever reach the point where I'm soiling my bed,
then please, take a shot gun and shoot me
before I get worse. Harsh words, I know,
but I saw too many people lying in hospital beds
that weren't people anymore. Just sticks with wrinkles
instead of skin, no hair, no teeth, some of them
with no arms or legs and no brain, sores
all over their bodies and pee and feces
pouring out at all hours. I'd hear them
sometimes groaning and weeping halfway down the hall
in another room, calling for their wives and mothers
with the nurses only stopping in every so often
to make sure they were sedated enough to sleep.
A lot of them once they came to the hospital
never went out again, except in a box.
But why am I telling you all this! You're young
and you got a family and the grass ain't brown yet.
I wish you a happy life. You're a nice young man.
Stop by to see me when you're out this way again.
You drive safely now."

WHATEVER IT TAKES

Erma is one of those patients who grumble and groan,
shake their head at every suggestion toward how to get better
and even spit out a four-letter word when she feels
like telling me what I can do with all the exercises
she needs to perform to reach a goal of walking
through her yard again to reach her daughter's house
across the road.

       "I know, I know, I did it just a month ago
and the family wants me to walk there for Thanksgiving. . .
But it don't make sense—why the hell did they buy me a wheelchair
if they demand that I use my own two legs!
People are damned funny at times, and even though
I fell twice getting into bed, I sure as hell didn't plan
to have physical therapy. My daughter and doctor
plotted that one!"

       "But therapy is only for your benefit," I say.
"Anything to help your walking and balance can't be bad."

"Sonny, I'm eighty-two years old and I don't need you
or the Baptist preacher down the street telling me what's good for me.
I've put in my time. I worked thirty-six years waiting tables
at a diner in Bristol, Tennessee, and only came up here
because my kids forced me to. I've used my legs
more than they were meant to be used. If I want to sit
and have someone roll me to a dinner party
then roll me back home, then I'm damn well entitled to it."

I bite my lip. Take a full breath. Nod. Smile.
"You're right, Erma, you can do as you wish.
No one can pull you out of that chair against your will.
But. . .what harm is there in strengthening your muscles a little?
What's bad about helping your ability to stand

and improve coordination? They're all good things!
You don't want to fall anymore, do you?"

She scowls. Stares out the window. "No. . .I don't want to fall.
Ever again." Her voice alters. "That's probably why
I stay glued to this chair." She looks back at me.
"I'm afraid. I've never had nobody help me before
and I don't want them to start having to help me
off the floor each time I miss the mattress.
Can't you understand that!"

                              "I do. But they're going
to have to help you even more each time you need
someone to wheel you to the grocery store
or haul you to the doctor's or the hospital."
My harshness shocks her. But sometimes
harshness is the only thing that works. "Erma, your muscles
will atrophy and your organs deteriorate
if you sit all the time. Our bodies are not made for sitting.
And I know you have it in you to stand and walk again.
These exercises can make your legs strong enough to do so.
But no one can do them for you. No one—but yourself."

There is a curse on the tip of her tongue, but instead
she eyes me sternly. "Sonny, part of me wants to believe you,
but part of me believes the Man above only gives us
so many days. If you think you got something over him
then. . . I'll do as you ask." She pauses, smiles, briefly,
for the first time, ever. A cagey smile.
"So, how many extra days do I get for each exercise?"

THE LAST VISIT

The farmhouse where Mrs. Reese lives with her husband of sixty years
lies on a road up a mountain paralleled by a stream
rushing over rocks in a series of mini-waterfalls.
This morning the water roars like thunder from weeks
of snowthaw, days of rain; ice on curves makes the drive
slower than usual. I take my time also to study the woods
soon to leaf out with green. I won't be coming back for awhile.
(If ever).
The old woman I've been treating for a month has decided
to accept her doctor's advice and go ahead
with a leg amputation at the knee. The infection on her calf
has not healed and will not heal, and a prosthesis appears
the safer option for future walking and livelihood.

Why did she even want one more visit?
Though, she has told me many times: "I always feel good
after I exercise and walk around the house with you to watch me.
I don't feel safe doing it with my husband
because he's as sick as I am. Sicker! He has more
doctor's appointments every year than birthday candles
on his cake. I don't think I would have said this at the start:
but I'm going to miss you coming up here.
Gave me something to look forward to. . ."

Of course there is the risk at her age of surgery,
let alone removing an entire limb. The surgeon
has told her of the risk, but she shrugs it off.
"I know honey, but as much pain as I've had the last
twenty or so years, death might be the better choice.
No matter what you or the doctor say."

I don't try to dissuade her. We can never gauge another's pain.

We can never prove whether one choice is truer than another.
We can never decide whether life is sweeter than death.

SNOWFLAKES IN A WARM HAND

LEGACY

For the first time since the funeral I stand
at the grave of my father. The wash of wind
has dropped acorns from the old oak that throws
shadows over the placement of his ashes.
It is a beautiful place to be buried.
An ancient cemetery with Revolutionary-era tombs no longer legible.
An even older church once frequented by George Washington.

I don't know why I haven't come earlier.
Four years, five years, I try not to count, feeling guilty
at lost time. I believe you would understand.
Working, supporting a family, the intentions
were always there to make the pilgrimage
but distractions are the bane of the world.
Excuses excuse us.
                    Though. . .wasn't it the same
with you and your father? I never saw his grave,
somewhere in Greenville, South Carolina.
You never drove us there on a sidetrip during vacations.
Why? The same guilt? The same hindrances of family and career?

Or was it something else? I never met my grandfather;
dead of emphysema before I was born. Only a few pictures
of a tall, slender, blond-haired man who always
stared at the camera with closed lips between a smile and a frown.
All I ever saw of him. And sadly it's the same with my two children.
Oh, they've seen pictures of you, but you left us
before they entered this oddity called life.
And they only have my words for descriptions.
Of your blunt jokes and savage temper
and the way you always liked to pay for huge dinner parties
to the chagrin of my mother.

I miss you.
But I can't say I miss you a lot. Not to the extent
of thinking of you every day. I'm not sure it's wise
to remember all the time. Not even the good things.
The acorns fall and soon the leaves will follow them.
Soon we all will follow them. And that is our legacy.

RECESSION

Outside the gates of the auto plant they sit.
Several dozen wrapped in large coats and scarves
warming themselves beside a bonfire.
A few hold signs stating, *We stand together.*
And, *Don't take our jobs, we have children too.*

They've been sitting there for two weeks.
Taking turns with others, shifting schedules,
some A.M., some P.M.
Wives bring them hotdogs and home-made soup.
Friends stop by with cigarettes and coffee
and boxes of doughnuts.

But it is cold. Already they've weathered three snowfalls.
Another is in the forecast tonight.
Tomorrow, sleet.

The first night a local station showed them on the news.
No reporters lately, though.
And no certainty the owners in Europe have even heard.
There's only the rumor of a closing date in April
and the entire plant moving overseas
to Bangladesh or Thailand.

They shake their fists and curse when a foreman
drives in and out of the gates.
But armed guards at the portal
keep them from doing more.

EVEN SAI BABA HAS TO TAKE A CRAP

A wait of five hours, the big screen relays.
I had taken the morning flight from Copenhagen to Heathrow
en route to Washington DC and now I have to sit
or walk or sleep or drink or eat or twiddle my thumbs in Terminal 3
until the British Airways jet is ready for boarding.

So I find a seat and pull out a book of quotes by the greatest philosophers
but can't scan more than a few lines
before noticing my seat lies directly in front of the bathrooms.

I put the book away and get up to move but. . .sit down again.
Two Hasidic Jews walk out of the bathroom while two Arabs
in robes and headdresses walk in. Then two little girls and their mother
come out. A Rastafarian passes by them going in.

This is more titillating than Kant or Aristotle. A beautiful blonde
speaking Swedish to a not-so-good-looking brunette
hurries in high heels toward the Ladies' room. A red-nosed fat man
walks out just after the girls are lost to view, sighing, much relieved.

This goes on for hours. A group of Japanese tourists
almost stampede past me; some sports team in blue outfits
(they speak a Slavic tongue) 15 minutes later do the same.

At one point I go to the bathroom myself. A man with a dot on his forehead
glances at me while washing his hands. A Catholic priest races by me
    to a stall.
There are the usual noises and smells; a dwarf-sized custodian
mops the floor. I look at my watch. Only an hour to go.
I return to the same seat. A slim redhead comes out just after me
and smiles. Two young men in white shirts and black ties
stop in front of me and ask if I'd be interested in reading

the Book of Mormon. I shake my head, then they too turn
to the toilet area. One of them comes out again promptly,
pulling up his zipper, the other takes ten minutes.
I feel like telling him:

If you want religion, just sit here awhile and observe.
This is the only religious book you'll ever need.

AND THE MORAL IS...

"They shot him down like a cur,
on a backstreet in Belfast. Not even IRA.
Shot him dead! He was a friend. A good friend..."
The little Irishman sat on the sofa opposite me,
beside him, an English couple, friends of mine.
I had eaten dinner with the couple: vegetable curry,
red wine, chocolate cake as dessert.
They had told me they expected their friend Cormac to come
but he was late, so we ate without him,
and while sleet drummed the windows
we spoke of our jobs and the weather
and current films we had yet to see
and our adjustment to an alien culture
(the three of us being voluntary exiles
in Denmark) and the long winter of Scandinavian dark.
With candles cozying out the gloom,
we sat and chatted for an hour or two
when finally there was a knocking on the door
and the Irishman stumbled in, Guinness-breath
strong and eyes reddened from drink, or tears, or both.

"They blew his head off," he mumbled
in some Northern Irish jargon.
"The bastards took him for a terrorist, and now he's gone."

Collapsing on the sofa he lay there half-crying, half-cursing,
while the three of us stared—tight-lipped in astonishment,
not knowing whether to ask questions or stay silent.
None of us had lost friends like that...
What could we say? Cormac eventually rose
to a sitting-position and wiped his tears on his shoulders.

"Would you like something to eat?" Helen asked.

Cormac looked at her blankly. "No. Just get me a beer.
And then get me another one. Tomorrow
I'm going back home—I'm joining up!"

For the rest of the evening we sat like stones.
Cormac finished three beers and was asleep
when I told my friends I'd be heading home.
They apologized for Cormac's behavior.
As I left, the footfalls of my steps
echoed across the five-story stairwell,
and I wondered why apologies
must always be said for the pained and drunk.
I wanted to go back and console him
                              but outside,
the sleet had become snow.
Bundling up, I focused on the cold
—and the long half-hour it would take
to walk the sloshy streets
in a sudden weariness, home.

JANUARY WIND

Walking beside this little creek in the foothills of the Blue Ridge
with my wife and children
hearing leaves dead for three months rustling
across forest in the January wind
I can't help but think once a squaw and her husband
and their children
tread this very path, anticipating spring
in the same way we do,
believing in life
that will always be
there.

THE MORE THINGS CHANGE THE MORE THINGS STAY THE. . .

Never once have I heard my daughter utter
a four-letter word, but tonight at dinner
she says, "Daddy, there are three girls
on my school-bus who use the F-word
in every sentence. One of them's pregnant!
And only thirteen!" Her words stun me
and I nearly drop my fork. Tia is eleven,
first year in Middle School, first year
riding a school-bus. I look at her. . .
Her eyes are as blue as they were when she was three.
Wasn't that only the day before yesterday?
She still giggles like a child now that the subject
has changed as she goofs off with my five year old son,
laughing at the way he slurps up spaghetti.
I'm about to say I don't like the way
the world is heading, the direction of youth
—but just a few decades earlier my parents
shook their heads at the same fallings,
teenagers sleeping together, marijuana,
the disrespect for authority. I thought
they were a couple of old farts, and now,
worried at other things Tia must soon encounter,
I wonder whether I'm one myself. . .

LUNCH AT THE MALL

It was a food court in Florida. My girl and I
had purchased jambalaya and Cajun rice
with chicken respectively when we heard
the commotion at another eatery. A shoving match.
Foul words. Something about the food tasting bad,
overpriced. A woman harangued a worker
while her boyfriend tussled with the manager
then security was called, and the couple involved
high-tailed it out of there. The place had been noisy
as a monkey pen; but during the fight: SILENCE.
Then just as suddenly patrons began to talk again,
as I found a table, one of the few left.

"Did you hear what that woman said?" a man asked
another man at the table beside ours.

I bit off a piece of stale cornbread as the other man answered:

"Yes. She said he was worse than Ted Bundy
and Jack the Ripper rolled into one, interspersed"—he laughs—
"with sex-with-mother connotations."

My girl and I sat there eating, silently, listening for awhile
as the others' conversation drifted toward football games
and problems with their spouses. I don't know why
we sat there so silent, not saying anything
as the rest of the room resumed garbled chatter,
though L— was the type who disliked useless talk
and I usually obliged her. In the meantime I imagined
the angry couple running from the mall,
jumping in their car, speeding off, cursing the incident
and cursing the world. Of course they could have been

getting ready to rob a bank or plotting to shoot the president. Regardless, they were *right* about the food:

BAD. . .and way overpriced.

THIS TALE'S BEEN TOLD BEFORE

It was chronicled that the Frankish King Clothair,
who conquered nearly all of Germany, Gaul, and Northern Spain,
and was a man who had murdered every rival to his throne,
in the winter of 561 AD on his death bed gasped
with his last breath of air: "Fate is cruel! And how great
the King of Heaven is who can kill kings
as powerful as I am." Then he died, and was buried,
and soon forgotten like all other kings before him.

EPICUREAN IN THE ORIGINAL SENSE

There are nights when frost throttles the ground
barely an hour after sunset, and the western horizon
blurs with fog and ice-storm, and I cannot help
but think the world will never again be warm.

And then you say: *Dinner is ready.*
And I tell the children and we come eager to the table.
Bowls of lentil soup await us. Hot wheat rolls
you've made yourself. We sit, and slurp the soup, slowly.

A beginning sleet, hail, slap the windows,
fist the roof. We listen, wondering how slick
the morning will be. Wondering whether snow
will cover the roads. Then each of us eats another bowl.

Soon, no rolls remain. We smile afterward, saying little.
No more noise outside. Only a white stream of endlessness, falling.

ONE FOOT IN FRONT OF THE OTHER

The dawn sun like a bloodred poppy
breathed high over sea and city
when I walked from my girl's apartment
to the nearest subway stop.
I was tired, and my body smelled of sweat
and love juice and spilled wine
but it was a happy-tired, and I was in love,
and spring had finally thawed the world
of Baltic cold.

As I approached the station
I saw blue cornflowers
strewn along the rail-lines.
But nearer the station an orange ribbon
cordoned off the entrance-way while police
and firemen
ran up and down the stairs.
Two ambulance drivers
hurried from the street bearing
a white-sheeted stretcher.
Somewhere there was sobbing and a voice
in half-sentence said: "—just like that!
He jumped in front of the train.
The driver had no time to do anything."

A crowd began to gather and gawk.
I watched as the ambulance-men returned
with some misshapened lump atop the stretcher.
Pushing it into their vehicle, they slammed
the doors, got in, turned the sirens on,
drove off.

A woman looked imploringly at a policeman:
"But I *work* at the next stop."
The officer shook his head. "You'll have
to take a bus or taxi. Or walk."

I rubbed my eyes.
It struck me all of a sudden
that a few hours ago
while I was making love
the victim might have been
beating nails into his skull.
The woman continued to beseech
the policeman. More fireman
entered the station.

I nudged through the crowd,
crossed the street, and felt
a few coins in my pocket.
Just enough for a bus.
Two blocks down was a bus stop
where a yellow bus pulled up.
I ran; a car honked, swerving
to avoid hitting me.
I was a block away when the bus
sped off. The next one wouldn't
come for twenty minutes.

I stood for a moment hearing the sirens
trail off in the city.
Across the lakes to the east
the spires of Copenhagen glinted with sunlight.
It would take an hour to walk home.
Or else wait for the next bus.
A police car raced past me.
I stepped one leg in front of the other
remembering the calm of twilight
not ten hours before
when my lover and I tread barefoot

by still-glacial strand-waters
watching kelp-clogged foams
thrown landward on blunt waves.
The blocks became mile markers
and each mile further
I walked faster, wanting to phone my girl,
to tell her what I forgotten to say at dawn
—what had seemed unnecessary
while we slept unawares that the world had altered.
Soon the street names became blurs
as the sun rose even higher.
After a while I heard no more sirens.

NOTHING MORE TO ADD

To Howard McCord

The swirls of sunset trail splashes in the west,
and the great painting of the sky is a mere instant.
Just an instant.
After that another instant.
After that. . .

Our error is seeing an instant more than an instant.
The universe is just a number. . .

WHO IS REALLY CAGED

My daughter's guinea pig *Sunny* is nearly five.
In the wild he'd be lucky to make one.
He steps lazily over the sawdust in his cage,
finds a carrot, chews it.
He's never known a life outside his cage.
Never heard the swoop of hawk wings
or the slither of a snake.
Most of us have scars, mental and physical,
but his brown fur is soft, his skin undamaged,
and he makes the same squeak when he's hungry
that he did when we first brought him home.

PATTERNS OR NOT

Overhead clouds darken as storm winds push across
the mountains to the east. Already October,
the geese seen last week in the light-lessened sky
must be half-way to their destination.
A curious thing, *Destiny,* or at least the definition
men give it. None of us know where we're headed,
or even if there is such meaning as direction.
We don't know what day birth greets us
or what day we'll die, and much of the time
we don't even know what we're eating for lunch.
The storm will come soon, and with it rain
colder than last month's rain, but not as cold
as the rain a month from now
—a year from now. . .

TYPICAL FACEBOOK ENTRIES

Sam Sterrow: I just took a good crap. Now I'm eating a pastry for breakfast with black coffee.

Jane Moogla: I can't decide whether I should go grocery shopping tonight or tomorrow.

Billy Slobber: After work I'm getting a six-pack of Bud and sitting down to watch THE BIGGEST LOSER.

Jane Moogla: I think I might go tomorrow. . .but I'm still not sure.

Ruth Lunk: It's Thursday—but God it feels like Monday. Must be the weather. Has anyone seen the forecast? It's supposed to rain the next three days!

Billy Slobber: Make that two six-packs.

Anthony Raisins: What are you complaining about, Ruth? In Burlington we've had ice and snow the past two weeks!

Jane Moogla: No, I've decided. I'll shop tonight.

Billy Slobber: And order a couple of extra large pizzas too. Or a calzone and one pizza.

Ruth Lunk: If you don't like Burlington, then move away.

Anthony Raisins: I didn't say I didn't like Burlington. I just said we've had snow and ice the past few weeks.

Jane Moogla: No no no, I'm shopping tomorrow.

Ruth Lunk: Well, I don't like rain or snow!

Anthony Raisins: Me either! But what's the sense in complaining about it. It's winter, baby.

Ruth Lunk: Anthony, you're butt-irritant.

Anthony Raisins: Is that even a word?

Sam Sterrow: I don't know if it's a word or not. But now I'm eating another pastry.

PLAYING CATCH

My seven-year old son is always asking questions.
Today we stand in the backyard throwing a football
and he asks, "Dad, why is everything made in China?
It says *Made in China* on this football
and they don't even play football in China!
And at school the other day I saw
a tiny American flag, and it was also *Made in China*."

I tell him it's cheaper to make things in China.

"But why?" he wants to know.

"Because here it costs too much to pay the workers,"
I explain. "The workers in China only get paid
a few pennies for their work. So it's easier
for the companies. They make more money that way."

"A few pennies!" He stops throwing the ball
and looks closely at it. "But how can they buy food?" he asks.
"They couldn't even buy this football for a few pennies."

"I know," I tell him. And nearly tell him that most of the world
can't buy a football. But he throws it again
without saying anything else. And I throw it back.

THE UNRETURNING

I often wonder whether the dead I've buried
might have altered the world, had they lived,
if only slightly. The childhood friend
who committed suicide by driving his Harley
into a brick wall at ninety-plus miles an hour
—He might have invented a motorcycle
that ran on ocean water.
And the girl I dated several months in college
who later drove off the side of a mountain
in a snowstorm with another boyfriend
—She might have become a state Senator
who put into effect a law requiring road lights
on every treacherous stretch of highway.
The guy I worked beside in the post office
who always smiled and never was sick
a single day I knew him then suddenly
one day was gone and no one knew where
until we heard a year later he had died of AIDS
—He might have written a bestseller
about how to stay happy while coping with disease.
I wonder about these early dead.
I wonder about the living who have time
but do so little with their lives.
We should all wonder.

SUMMER JOB

We'd been bearing bags of cow manure and peat moss
to the back of the nursery for two hours without stop
when Gill suddenly growled out: "I quit!
I can't take this crap job anymore.
They're treating us like slaves!"
And he made off toward the office, leaving
the rest of us there on the edge of the pasture.

He looked like a blob of dirt limping up the hill.
A bag of manure had split open and soiled his shirt,
black peat caked his legs and shoes,
sweat poured down his face and being heavy,
he guzzled breaths as though air was beer.

When he was out of sight, Tad said, "He's only
been here two days. What's his problem?"

All of us knew the answer. All of us being college boys
not used to tough labor, but surviving nonetheless.
A three month job, and not the best pay,
but a job regardless, it would keep us in shape.

So we returned to hauling the fifty pound bags,
stacking them in neat piles for the big weekend
sale.

AT THE END

It never fails. Whenever I feel despondent
or the mass culture of the world
rips my sanity with daggers
stained by greed, cruelty, conquest,
I'll go outside to watch the sunset
fastly fade; purple streams of light
so beautiful, the west horizon
a mass of orange-red swirls
meshing with dusk's darkening blues
on silhouettes of mountains
crowned with clouds.
Nature no more enduring
than news-flashes endears the mind
to the ephemeral values of our lives
and the life of the universe.
That no matter how rich or embracing
a moment is, how cut-throat or crushing:
None of it lingers. None of it lasts.
No pain eternal. No love infinite.
At the end—we are all sunsets,
and our murky lives come clear.

THIS IS THE TIME TO LOVE

The body the farmer found in his field at noon
was there when we embraced last night
in a fire of needs; was sprawled there when we stroked
and cuddled one another once the fires released
in sudden octaves; grew hard as steel
there when pinesap and grasses froze three hours
before dawn; lay still there when you nudged me
in the morning, smiling, and whispering:
You'll be late for work.

THE UNSTANDARD

If you're looking for a creed to follow,
a standard planted and established by men
who have long been dust but left rules to govern
your humanity under a singular oath,
a cement culling the multitude into believing as one,
then listen for awhile, and I'll tell you
without jingoism that all that is human
is no longer human for it is too human.
Ours saturates the universe where there are
no other voices allowed. The lion has no say,
neither the penguin nor the millipede,
neither the alder or savanna grass,
quarry stone, or labradorite.
And the *few* who speak for them. . .are considered
crackpots or worse. Remember this if you remember anything:
The power-mongers and preachers want to muffle the mind
and keep it muffled; the mob is never encouraged to stand alone.
But you can *only* ever stand on a mountaintop alone;
no one can stand there for you.
If you want to be a free-thinker then free yourself
from all thinking besides your own.
Re-learn instinct. Re-learn to live like wind and water
that never become entrapped by anything.
Walk away from what disgusts and disenchants you,
but if forced to fight then fight fiercely
like a badger cornered. Trust no human theory completely.
Not even your own, unless it allows you to wander
and allows others to wander too.

CYNICISM FOR DUMMIES

The latest mass murder in the news brings the usual array
of mourners placing wreathes and bouquets
atop the shooting site, and reporters and journalists
asking the oft-repeated lines: "Why? What caused this
to happen? Have we not learned from previous tragedies?"

But should we really be surprised that history turns the same page
and we rarely learn from it. New generations come along
and think they're invincible; new Gavrilo Princeps wait in ambush
to set the fuse to wars and race-hatred; new doom-Sayers
stamp words on minds deranged with unfulfillment.

The real surprise is that we seek answers where there never were any.
We question events that no animal would ever question,
simply because we have forgotten that every day is new,
and the world never locks its eyes on a single story,
for nothing is a story.

NO BIGGER THAN A SHOE BOX

Mid-day, but mid-day in Denmark in February
is nearer to dark, a darkness summer never knows.
Patches of snow on the ground; wind and rain
scratching skin like cat claws; cold, borne
inland from the Baltic. All of us, the twenty

or so people huddled in coats and scarves
listening to a priest: one of the psalms,
one of the sermons to give solace to the living
and final declaration to the dead.
My wife's grandmother, for ten years an invalid,

speechless, drooling, legless, lying under woolen blankets
even in July—now returned to the world
of the unborn and the dead in an urn
no bigger than a shoe box, no wider than a hand.
Have I found a perfect tone for a poem?

Sacred, solemn, the painful solitude
of each person standing in the group
though alone, thoughts of death, of parting,
sundered only by need to flee the freezing minutes.
Yet what is haunting in something that happens

every hour of every day in every nation
on every atoll, island and continent?
All the non-newsworthy tragedies
that never flood the headlines but strike horror in the hearts
of specific families and friends.

In this instance a woman who'd come of age
during the Depression, poor, married young,

bore two children amongst the German Occupation,
made her husband dinner every night for forty years
and was shouted at and hit for spending too much on groceries,

gave candy to her grandchildren (secretly),
enjoyed holidays, then grew ill: cancer,
dementia, gangrene, amputation. . .*death.*
The priest's words end, and my wife's eyes
streak with tears—I want to kiss them away,

hold her, let her bury her head on my chest.
But these people are Vikings, hugging is rare,
and tears rarer. An indentation
in the hard soil is all that remains.
And later a reception at a cheap café.

TIGER'S PAW

The sunset's a tiger's paw clawing west across the blue range of mountains,
scraping furrows of light on green corn fields and valleys.
I have seen many beautiful sunsets in forty-some years,
none exactly the same; in fact, have there ever been two sunsets
on the earth exactly the same? The silliness of sacred texts
stating the divine power of the universe is a rock
that never alters shape or meaning—when everything
everywhere is constant change!
                      Maybe I better halt
before my own words brand me. Men I suppose need
their creeds because *Change* is a curve-ball that strikes them out every time.
But the sky is so beautiful: purple, orange, red, blue,
a forge of torching fire unheld by human hands,
harnessed to no other drama than its own momentary hymn
played before no paying audience.
                       Beauty? Truth? It may
be these things or it may not be. Soon it will be gone.
Just like everything else.

PROLONG

Today my eleven year old daughter asks me
why there is war in the world, whether
I believe in God, and whether there is life
after death. I look at her. Yesterday
she decorated doll houses and surrounded
her bed with cuddly hippos. . .and now. . .

Like too many others I spend daily hours
working for some corporate monstrosity
that could care less about important questions
and even less so about me. Only MONEY
drives the interest of our culture, politicians, media,
religions. Some might say otherwise, but. . .

Few of us can choose from anything but one menu.
Daughter, I want to hold you in the gaze of my eyes forever,
just as you are, not the adult you are to become.
I know it is foolish, and the vague answers
I give your questions are silly attempts to prolong
your childhood. Rather let me say I hope

your life is a lovely dance, that you enrich
yourself with simplicity and find love by loving,
that you meet a man who flies with the same wings,
that you always have friends, that you understand
how short/beautiful life is and how all answers must be your own.
Mostly. . .I hope the headlines of the world never need you for a story.

YOU CAN NEVER STEP INTO THE SAME RIVER TWICE

A friend of mine bemoans the fact that he traveled
to India as a young man and now having just gone
there again with a wife and three children
finds the place altered, more commercial,
teeming with street vendors and pickpockets
and well. . .not the same. . .

But places are rarely the same when you visit them later,
whether the Big Sur coast, the Analects of Confucius,
or the body of your fourth lover,
they have all changed, or rather you have changed
and cannot see them the same way you did
twenty, thirty years ago. *So why even try?*

And that's what I told him. Act like it's a new country
you're journeying to, neither horror nor oasis.
Just an exotic roundabout you learned of
from someone you once knew. . .

THE FACTS OF LIFE

Some, are just favored by the gods;
others are the dung beetles
of the universe.

RUPERT BROOKE'S GHOST

Ah! I hear a voice. It calls me out of the murk
of the undefined. It claims a part of my lifelessness
to arise and give earnest answers. Who are you,
to beg from the marrow of bones a torch unlightable?

Another fancier of words. Another framer of verse.
A man that finds worth in lost poets. I seek
to query you for the hoard that was too young entombed.

Well, query away then. My mouth has been filled
with ashes too long, and my body bears the verdict
of an exile never to be overturned.

I will be blunt. And quick.
What do you miss most about the world? About Life?

Do I need to answer! Walking bare feet on morning dew.
Women, my God women! Wine, good ale, a savory pot
of stew. Dawn over a grove of coconut trees.
Writing a sonnet to a lover. Kissing her lips, hair, breasts.
Watching a storm by candlelight.
Oh, just to be alive!

But you have gained the immortality you longed for in a poem. . .

Indeed. . .immortality! Alone, lying here on a Greek isle
in the Aegean. Nothing but sea, sun and earth for companions.
But I don't feel the same now. Looking back,
I see the war was such an awful waste. All those men
bleeding out their youth and lives—*for what?*
So that another war could happen twenty years later!
Then more wars after that. Yes, I've gained an ivory tower

in death, though what does that mean to a man
who only wants life, love, the unlimited mead of youth. . .

But dying unold has always been romantic;
did you not say so yourself? Is your grave
not forever a part of England—as you wished?

We all say silly words in our lives. Unfortunate words.
I would take them from the anthologies if I could.
If it meant bright blood thrilled my veins again
and my skin could once more chill to a rain
in Warwickshire, then I would utter that I had never
uttered them. In this place where the cold
does not even chill and is beyond poetical description,
and the darkness is a darkness that has
no counterpart in light, my eyes are finally opened
to see clearly what cannot be seen when breath
fills the lungs. If I had been one man dying
for the homeland then my barrow would rival
Lord Byron's in Missolonghi; the rows of mounds
in Flanders and Gallipoli altered the perception
that dying for King and Country is the ultimate epitaph
for a soldier. We were wronged! The whole generation
was horribly wronged, mutilated, misled,
shoved out of the way of the next generation
and buried even when alive, so that the tortured voices
were always only a few. Might I have become
one of those voices. . .O, I cannot imagine otherwise.
I cannot imagine losing a life for a cause ignoble
to the individual, for a culture that maims
through patriotism its singular sons.

Your speech trembles. I fear I have awoken you unjustly.
May I ask another question? One more?

Perhaps I have said enough. The jaw aches
after having spoken nothing for a century.
What is it you wish?

Would you fight those in power who started the war?
Would you tell others that peace is the only flag worth raising?

You ask of me conduct that was written impassioned
well after the last dirt was thrown on my coffin.
Pacifism. . .that runt of the litter rarely had strength
to run when I and my comrades shouldered our rifles
and boated to France. Few in Europe or the world
at that time found honor in peace. Cowardice,
we equated with those too weak-limbed
and brittle-minded to share the load
in halting the Hun. We were honeyed by the hour
with slogans of duty, integrity, and revenging
Belgian children. We were slammed with the sledgehammer
of hating all the enemy stood for, their annihilation
of small nations, their desecration of virtues
creeded in the marble of Athens. Oddly, does not the same
even occur now? Are foes not described as maggots
and serving one's ancestral home believed
the highest wreath after worshiping God?
In many ways your era is worse than ours.
For you have weapons to massacre the whole earth
while we were barely beyond mounting cavalry charges.
And I can't say I think much of your men of verse.
Or women of verse. Your lines are less pretty,
and your subject matter is a bore. May I go?
What else must I answer, if I even choose to. . .

Nothing. Nothing more. I'm sorry I woke you.
The dead can't answer for the living.
And I've been a fool to think they could.
Only the living can do that.
If they only will.

123

GOODNESS

More than a word, goodness is a genre with few above it.
But often I close the door on its open hands and lock
myself into a world of thought, not noticing that all the while
you have kept the kitchen clean, the house, a husband
happy, a daughter and son cared for—and go to work without complaint.
Yes I neglect your benedictions like an arrogant king
who has forgotten who filled his grail, lost sight
of your benevolence, the tokens of your love-notes
and even now, the sweet peas and cosmos
you have placed on my desk. Wife, you are more than good,
and when my selfish moments of writing writing writing
dull like a worn ring
I see it more and more. I see that time and life and love
fall away into severless winter and the words that rune
the bulk of my essence bear poor witness in comparison
to one sign of your heart. Your goodness is an open diary
without secrets, and our moments so few
to build steeples to joy.

AND IN SPACE IT DOESN'T EVEN RAIN

The rain that falls on the graves at Gettysburg is the same rain
that falls on the nearby fields of corn, the same rain
that falls on the streets of Paris and the people-less taiga of Siberia,
that falls on tigers in India on mosquitoes in Alaska,
on redwood forests on prairies on jungles on sand grains in the Gobi,
on child molesters on missionaries on castles on slums
on unemployed on CEOs on pacifists on generals
on Israel on Palestine
on oceans on creeks
on Christians on Atheists
on democrats on republicans
on astrophysicists on plumbers
on poets on dishwashers
on prisoners on prison wardens
on men on women
on toddlers on elderly with Alzheimer's
on happily married on recently divorced
on suiciders on newborn
on high school valedictorians on high school drop outs
on fisherman on netted fish
on murder victims on murderers
on socially adapted on schizophrenics
on football players on deaf and blind
on me, and on you
the same rain
the same rain.

EARTH JOY

The lettuce seeds barely a week under ground already sprout,
and the arugula shows green too.
A robin gathers twigs in its beak; honeybees swarm dandelions,
     lilacs, clovers.
There is not a cloud in the sky, and the purple clusters
of redbuds paint the mountains. I am amazed
how spring never ceases to come no matter
what people do to the earth or what gods we believe in
or don't believe in. I am in awe how the world
doesn't need us, and never has. With such beauty in the land,
the red dust of history disappears. I think Tao Chien knew this
when he turned his back on Imperial China
to sow millet and plant plum trees
and write poems that no one in his time ever read.

PHILODEMUS REFLECTING ON THE DEATH OF CASSIUS

When he heard the news that Cassius had died by his own hand
after losing the fight at Philippi, Philodemus
left his house at Herculaneum to muse along the sea.
To the north Mt. Vesuvius hovered over the land,
westward the waters of the Gulf of Naples
blue beneath a cloudless sky. Besides a few farmers
steering oxen in a field, a man driving a wagon
of clay pots to town, the world was windless,
the world was quiet.

Philodemus had chosen this spot precisely for the quiet,
the peace his Epicurean nature found far from Rome
and other noisy cities. Poems came in abundance
on this beautiful coast. Pupils had called on him
from afar to learn his hexameters. Virgil,
Lucretius, Horace, even Cicero. Caesar's
father-in-law, Piso—he'd considered a good friend.

And Cassius, too. Though the murder of Julius Caesar
had shocked not only Rome but those who shared little
contact with Rome. Cassius. . .a man who named
himself an Epicurean, supposedly with a need
for solace and connections without turbulence,
had performed a deed Epicurus would never
have condoned—no matter the circumstances.
If the world smells like a latrine and men
wallow in its manure then step off the mired road
and build a garden far from the corrosion.
Entertain friends there, eat frugal meals, make
kindness your religion and simplicity your creed.

Any other demands are not those of Epicurus.

But Cassius—it must be remembered the man was a Roman
and not a Greek—justified killing Caesar
on grounds a tyrant posed absolute danger
to human serenity. In other words, he believed
Epicurus—who had never known the Romans—
would sanction the death of one villain
for communal safety, national well-being.

Philodemus shook his head. *I also am a Greek,* he thought.
Having lived among the Romans so long now. . .
perhaps I have overlooked the traits that give the lion its mane.
A mind wrinkled from years of habits
does not suddenly become smooth
at a few words of bliss. He stared at the waves
that never stopped breaking on the shore.
The lions were roaring again to the east.
The victors at Philippi bearing fangs at one another.
And tomorrow the new victors feeling fangs
of younger lions. What role does philosophy
play in any of this? Philodemus saw the man
returning from town with an empty wagon.
The farmers still plowed the field.
The mountain still hovered in the sky
and the sea was still sea. Here the world
was windless, the world quiet. He smiled.
Why had he been foolish to think otherwise. . .

IS THIS THE REASON WE BUILD
MONUMENTS AND PUT NAMES ON THEM

Here in the middle of December I stand on a hill-trail
wondering at the silence of this forest, the large oaks
their branches and bark gray as sky, the hemlocks
and pines their needles green with no competition.
Small crystals of snow drop to the leaf-brown earth
and on nearby streams, fading as quietly as they fall.

I am humbled to admit my presence is not needed
and will never be needed anywhere in these woods.
No human presence needed. The wind carries
no name with it except wind. Snow whitens ground
and it is only snow. I yell out into the vastness
and the echo of my voice makes the silence silenter.
My tracks on the ground already begin to fill. . .

THE WORLD ACROSS THE STREET

She died alone one autumn after I had gone
to college; divorced, no companions
besides two dachshunds, Mrs. Belk:
neighborhood mystery, rarely seen,
never employed, rumored a drug addict
and drunkard, who cussed out the paper boy
for being late and threatened to shoot
a traveling salesman soliciting hairspray
was found in her bedroom by a cousin
three days after her demise. *A strange bird*,
the young couple who lived next door said.
As kids we'd always thought her a witch
with her pasty white skin and long
black hair, the stare that would immobilize
you whenever she stood at the open front door
to make certain you weren't stepping
in her yard. The only time I ever heard
her speak—four of us teased her dogs
from the woods beyond her fence
when she burst out of the house
shaking fists at us: *Leave those dogs alone!*
Get the hell away from that fence!
After initial shock, being teenagers, we
strolled away with surly looks, but inside
we were shaking. *That bitch is scary*, Sean commented,
then we thought no more of it. I learned
later that the cousin took the dachshunds,
while the ex-husband inherited the house.
He let it sit there for six months, before
selling it to a family from El Salvador,
who held a noisy barbecue
every Saturday night in the summer.

130

CASTLES OF SAND

With you I never thought we'd run out of a west to find,
or a north, south, east. If there weren't roads
we'd have paved our own. If mountain passes were blocked
we'd have found a way through them.
Fate was with us like a sun that never set.

But suns do set, and so do people and dreams.
And no poems, prayers, tears, bring them back.

DOING THE BEST I CAN

It's no doubt happened twenty billion times,
sitting down to write, inspired, the words firing
out of me like tommy gun bullets

—then. . .

an interruption. My son kicking a ball against a door,
my daughter yelling for me from another room,
asking whether she can have a sleep-over next Saturday,
my wife turning on the washer-and-dryer,
the telephone ringing and the door-bell ringing
and a car swerving around the corner outside,
tires screeching on a wet street.

It could be worse, I could be trying to put my thoughts down
on a piece of mud-spattered paper in a frozen fox-hole
with frozen fingers in some forgotten war half-way across the globe,
only to drop my pencil in the darkness
and watch the paper blow away in the wind.

GENERAL TSO'S CHICKEN

The night my girl and my best friend joined me for a meal
at a local Chinese restaurant outside Copenhagen
we ate and drank like we hadn't had real food in ten days
and then the fireworks started. . .our waiter,
who we thought from the beginning was either
a little stoned or drunk or a mixture of both
suddenly brought us more dishes that we hadn't ordered.

Then on being rebuked, he took them to other tables
with the same results. Eventually he took them back
to the kitchen. And returned with more trays full
of Lo mein and General Tso's chicken, though
we hadn't ordered them and no one else had
anywhere near us. We watched, began to laugh. Madly.
People gave the waiter dirty looks, and gave us
dirty looks too. My girl, amused tears rolling down
her cheeks, turned fearful when the manager appeared.

But he said nothing to us, only screamed at the waiter,
who putting the trays down on an unused table,
took out a bill and gave it to a man who had just
entered the restaurant.
                    "You have to pay for your food!"
the waiter said to the man.
                    "But I just walked in,"
the man answered, looking scared and confused.

"No, you didn't," the waiter replied.
"You're trying to leave without paying."

"But I tell you—I just got here!"
The man was even more frightened.

Other people started yelling for their bills.
Some people just got up and left.

The manager looked like he was having a stroke.

We kept on laughing, and the waiter brought us
ice cream we also had not ordered.
We kept on laughing, even after we paid
and left the place.

CONTACT ME IF YOU KNOW
SOMETHING MORE

I think everyone wants to believe there is life after this one,
where we greet our lost loved ones in some Tir Na Nog
of total serenity without drama. . .
But the salmon I eat tonight—will it return one day as the same salmon
to a heaven of clear, cold streams and passive ocean?
The rice and broccoli. . .will they too reforge in the same forms?

In these cases doubt outweighs belief. And the ashes of my Father,
that we buried in the Falls Church graveyard, will they ever
reconstruct into the molecular configurations
that laughed, yelled, snored, and cursed in a way like no other. . .

Silly questions, I know; Pythagoras couldn't answer them
and neither Einstein nor the cashier at the grocery store
comfort the mind with iron-hard knowledge
that individual consciousness is eternal. . .
Snowflakes falling in a warm hand. The only answer
the universe gives us.

CPSIA information can be obtained at www.ICGtesting.com
Printed in the USA
BVOW010454281112

306639BV00001B/26/P